Living

a

Lighter

Lifestyle

D1530632

Living a Lighter Lifestyle

A Guide to Successful Weight Loss and Maintenance Following Weight Loss Surgery

FIFTH EDITION

GAYE ANDREWS PH D, LMFT

WHEAT FIELD PUBLICATIONS
109 Kiwi Court
Lincoln, CA 95648

This book is dedicated to the courageous men and women who have chosen weight loss surgery as a tool for a healthier, happier life.

Contents

Illustrations

Forward

Jann L. Holwick, MD, FACS
Diplomate American Board Of Surgery

From the earliest operations performed for the treatment of severe obesity, now decades ago, to the 1991 National Institutes of Health consensus statement endorsing gastroplasty and gastric bypass as valid surgical procedures, patients and surgeons have faced an arduous journey of refinement and acceptance not yet concluded. Support and understanding by our medical and many surgical colleagues lags woefully behind the assent "out of darkness" most of our patients have taken, due, in part, to adverse outcomes experienced by many small bowel bypass patients. Unfortunately, as members of the human race, many physicians remain prejudiced with regards to the severely obese, hold fast to the false value of dieting for such patients, fear unreal surgical dangers, and are unaware of the "state of the art." This is understandable, for, although the literature is replete with up-to-date articles and texts, they are with rare exception buried in the surgical, not general medical, sources.

Yet, even in current and comprehensive medical sources, the psychological profile and perioperative care of the mental well-being, challenges and recovery issues—all crucial to the ultimate overall success of our patients—is, with rare exception, given only token passing mention. The tacit message is that severely obese patients carry weight as a symptom of underlying psychological turmoil, but the ways and means of grappling with these causal disorders are rarely addressed beyond the recognition of need, and often relegated the tabloid-like stigma of day-time talk show topics. When my patients ask for sources of relevant literature, I have little more than technical articles to offer them from my files. Dr. Andrews' book is certainly a welcome addition to begin filling the void between medical science and the patient.

Although vertical gastroplasties offer the best weight-loss track record for the least amount of surgical and metabolic risk incurred, gastric bypass will increase the percent of success stories for "all comers." It is without question the procedure of choice for those identified preoperatively as sweet eaters and high-calorie snackers, and for most patients needing a second "revision" surgery. Dr. Andrews' psychological owners' manual is invaluable for all bariatric surgery patients, regardless of their procedure.

As we have always stressed to our mutual patients, any surgical procedure for weight reduction and control is only a tool—to be used properly by choice and effort—and all credit for success goes ultimately to them. Many have realized, retrospectively, that the first step—having the surgery—was actually the easiest. The new-found freedom of buying "off the rack" does not equate with the freedom from psychological problems unmasked by a new relative thinness. Unfortunately, a minority of our patients nation-wide avail themselves of the complete program (dietary, behavior modification, counseling, physical therapy, etc.) even when offered, though many have a feeling of security, and perhaps some increased element of success thereby, just knowing it is there. With Dr. Andrews available, our patients had no excuse short of extreme distance—sometimes not even that. She has gone more than the few extra 100 miles, literally, to see to the mental well-being of those entrusting their lives to our care. Her book is a welcome, concise, accurate, supportive, and much needed pocket advisor and friend for those initially considering gastroplasty or gastric bypass or moving forward after their surgery. Considering the source, I'm not surprised. Dr. Andrews has always impressed me with her seemingly effortless ability to give the gift of acknowledgment as a worthy individual to those with whom she interacts. One always feels better for the time spent with her. On behalf of past and future patients, thanks! ∾

Author's Preface

For over twenty years I have been a member of several teams of professionals dedicated to helping people who are severely obese improve their health and overall quality of life by having weight loss surgery. It is difficult to put into words what this opportunity has meant to me. The professionals with whom I work are caring, conscientious, and competent. The patients are courageous, persevering, and generally remarkable. I feel the work and the people enrich my life much more than I am able to enrich the work and the people in return.

After several years of being urged by patients to turn my patient education and support group materials into a book, I wrote *Living a Lighter Lifestyle*. It has been gratifying to share this work with thousands of professionals and patients across the United States and indeed, around the world. Because the field of weight loss surgery is ever growing and changing, I revise *Living a Lighter Lifestyle* as new surgeries, surgical methods, and lifestyle information becomes available. This fifth edition provides updated information on obesity and the various surgical procedures used as treatment.

As always, I hope *Living a Lighter Lifestyle* assists patients having weight loss surgery to achieve and maintain a healthier body weight. I also hope it helps family members and friends of patients having surgery to understand the benefits of weight loss surgery and how to support the patient toward his or her weight and health goals. Finally, I want those considering weight loss surgery to have an understanding of the procedures and the lifestyle adjustments necessary for success so that that they can make an informed decision about the value of the procedures for themselves. ∾

Acknowledgements

I tell patients that successful weight loss and maintenance following weight loss surgery is a team effort. They need the help of a skilled surgeon, hospital medical staff, support team members, and family and friends. No one can do it alone. That is true about writing a book, as well. There are people who helped me through the process of writing *Living a Lighter Lifestyle*. They deserve special recognition and appreciation. I would like to take this opportunity to thank them.

Gene Wytrykus, my ever-supportive husband.

Breanna, Kathy, Kimberly, Mindy, Robert, Roy; patients who contributed their personal experiences with weight loss surgery.

Sally Myers and Patti Pedrick, Registered Dietitians who provided invaluable consultation regarding dietary issues.

Diane LeMont, PH D and *Summer Perry,* PH D, MFT, colleagues who's collaboration always inspires.

Marc McNaughton, the Graphic Designer who provided the creative vision for the project.

And special thanks to... the many physicians, nurses, dietitians, and weight loss surgery program and hospital staff members that use *Living a Lighter Lifestyle* in their work with weight loss surgery patients. ∽

Part One

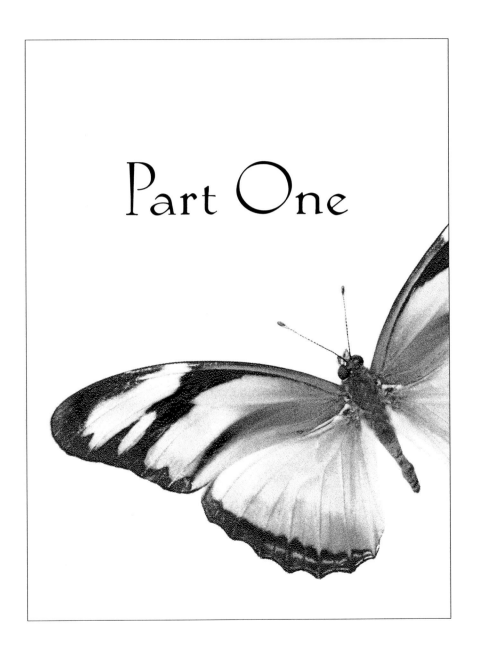

Kimberly

On my 34th birthday I took a step that was to be the turning point of my life. On that day, I had gastric bypass surgery.

Just a few days before, a million thoughts raced through my head and I asked myself many questions. Does it really have to come to this? Have I really done all that I can? How well will it work? What if I don't wake up from surgery? What if I do wake up and nothing changes?

When I was able to take a breath and slow my brain down, I was sure having gastric bypass was the right thing to do. I had been fat since I was about 3 years old. I had never known what it was to be "normal." I had negative, hateful feelings about myself and did not think I could go on with my life if I continued to be fat.

And I really had tried to lose weight through traditional dieting. Four years before, at my highest weight of 334 pounds, a family friend introduced me to a doctor who helped me lose 130 pounds in just over a year. It was great! Unfortunately, as with every other diet, I was not able to sustain the weight loss. I felt doomed like most people who lose hundreds of pounds only to regain them again, and then some.

The turning point for me was being faced with having to buy another size larger jeans. I was still not up to the size 28 or 30 I had worn before, but was terrified I would get there sooner or later. In an act of desperation, I called a bariatric surgery program I saw advertised on television. I had always thought

*that bariatric surgery programs were just a scam and that the
people who worked at "these programs" only cared about the
money, not the people who called. Boy was I wrong!*

*The first time I called, I asked about 1000 questions related
to gastric bypass surgery. Every one of them was answered. I
was offered a personal consultation appointment, but refused
saying I would call in a few weeks when things calmed down
at work. Two weeks later I made my second call and accepted
a consultation appointment a few days after that. I had my
surgery on April 30, 1998.*

*It's 8½ months after my surgery and I have lost 100 lbs. I
have about 45 pound more to go to achieve my goal. Because
of the surgery, I know I will reach my goal and this time, I
will not gain it back. I have the strength to face the bad feelings and memories that I carried along with the excess weight
for so many years.*

*I feel that I now have a future and I would do the surgery
all over again in a heartbeat. Although the surgery was difficult and I did have some complications, in retrospect they
were nothing compared to the complications that 30 years of
being fat and hating myself had brought to my life.*

*I am often asked if I am proud of myself for having gastric
bypass. The truth? I am! And I am, honestly, just very thankful. Thankful that God has blessed me with this opportunity
and thankful for finding a program with wonderful, caring,
and truly supportive people.* ∾

CHAPTER ONE

Obesity: Causes, Effects and Treatment

In the United States about 25 percent of men and 40 percent of women are on a diet at any one time. Through medically supervised diet programs, commercially operated programs, or fad diets, these people are earnestly trying to lose weight. Research indicates that the success dieters experience varies greatly depending on starting weight, diet method, and length of diet. Some dieters do achieve and maintain a reduced body weight—although not necessarily their goal weight. The majority of dieters regain all of the weight they lost—and sometimes even more—within two to five years.

For unsuccessful dieters, each pound regained will take its toll in personal frustration and a sense of failure. For the severely obese the toll of those regained pounds may be especially high. Those excess pounds may lead to poor physical health, psychological distress, social prejudice and isolation, and economic discrimination.

Because of the failure of most diet programs to bring about permanent weight loss and because of the serious physical, psychological, social, and economic consequences of severe obesity, physicians have been working to develop diet programs that really work. Their efforts have led to the development of a number of surgical techniques designed to limit food consumption or absorption in order to facilitate weight loss. According to the American Society for Metabolic and Bariatric Surgery, there are currently three types of surgical procedures done to promote weight loss. These are the restrictive procedures, the combined restrictive and malabsorptive procedures, and the malabsorptive procedures. In addition to the three types of surgical procedures there are two methods of performing them. These are the "open" method and the "laparoscopic" method.

This guide is for those who are severely obese... those who are considering or have chosen to have one of the various surgical procedures as a means to achieve and maintain a healthier body weight. Those who are in need and deserving of a chance for a healthy body, a positive self-esteem, social comfort, economic opportunity, and an overall enriched quality of life. This guide will define severe obesity, its causes and effects. It will describe the various weight loss surgical procedures and how and why they work. It will present the lifestyle necessary for successful weight loss and maintenance following the procedures. (For simplicity the procedures will be referred to as weight loss surgery or surgeries.)

OBESITY: ITS CAUSES AND EFFECTS...

'Overweight' is defined as an excess body weight. Muscle, bone, fat and/or body water may contribute to excess weight. Obesity is defined as an excess of body fat. From a medical perspective, those who are obese are suffering from a kind of physical illness or, at the very least, they are at increased risk for developing an illness.

The most common method used to determine if obesity increases health risk is the body mass index (BMI). BMI is a calculation based on height and weight (weight in kilograms divided by height in meters squared). Charts have been developed as quick BMI references. A sample BMI chart is found in Table 1. A person is considered mildly obese if their BMI is 30.0 to 34.9, moderately obese if their BMI is 35.0 to 39.9 and severely obese if their BMI is 40.0 or above.

Body Weight *(pounds)*

Obesity:
Its Causes
and Effects...

Height (inches)	30	31	32	33	34	35	36	37	38	39	40	41	42	43	44	45	46	47	48	49	50	51	52	53	54
58	143	148	153	158	162	167	172	177	181	186	191	196	201	205	210	215	220	224	229	234	239	244	248	253	258
59	148	153	158	163	168	173	178	183	188	193	198	203	208	212	217	222	227	232	237	242	247	252	257	262	267
60	153	158	163	168	174	179	184	189	194	199	204	209	215	220	225	230	235	240	245	250	255	261	266	271	276
61	158	164	169	174	180	185	190	195	201	206	211	217	222	227	232	238	243	248	254	259	264	269	275	280	285
62	164	169	175	180	186	191	196	202	207	213	218	224	229	235	240	246	251	256	262	267	273	278	284	289	295
63	169	175	180	186	191	197	203	208	214	220	225	231	237	242	248	254	259	265	270	278	282	287	293	299	304
64	174	180	186	192	197	204	210	216	222	227	232	238	244	250	256	262	267	273	279	285	291	296	302	308	314
65	180	186	192	198	204	210	216	222	228	234	240	246	252	258	264	270	276	282	288	294	300	306	312	318	324
66	186	192	198	204	210	216	223	229	235	241	247	253	260	266	272	278	284	291	297	303	309	315	322	328	334
67	191	198	204	211	217	223	230	236	242	249	255	261	268	274	280	287	293	299	306	312	319	325	331	338	344
68	197	203	210	216	223	230	236	243	249	256	262	269	276	282	289	295	302	308	315	322	328	335	341	348	354
69	203	209	216	223	230	236	243	250	257	263	270	277	284	291	297	304	311	318	324	331	338	345	351	358	365
70	209	216	222	229	236	243	250	257	264	271	278	285	292	299	306	313	320	327	334	341	348	355	362	369	376
71	215	222	229	236	243	250	257	265	272	279	286	293	301	308	315	322	329	338	343	351	358	365	372	379	386
72	221	228	235	242	250	258	265	272	279	287	294	302	309	316	324	331	338	346	353	361	368	375	383	390	397
73	227	235	242	250	257	265	272	280	288	295	302	310	318	325	333	340	348	355	363	371	378	386	393	401	408
74	233	241	249	256	264	272	280	287	295	303	311	319	326	334	342	350	358	365	373	381	389	396	404	412	420
75	240	248	256	264	272	279	287	295	303	311	319	327	335	343	351	359	367	375	383	391	399	407	415	423	431
76	246	254	263	271	279	287	295	304	312	320	328	336	344	353	361	369	377	385	394	402	410	418	426	435	443
BMI > 30	30	31	32	33	34	35	36	37	38	39	40	41	42	43	44	45	46	47	48	49	50	51	52	53	54

Obese (BMI 30–39)   *Extreme Obesity* (BMI 40–54)

Table 1 – *A Sample Body Mass Index (BMI) Chart*

According to the Center for Disease Control (CDC), the incidence of obesity in the United States has increased over time. Nearly one-third of adults over the age of twenty have a BMI of or higher than 30. In the past thirty years the rate of obesity has nearly tripled for children (ages two to five) and adolescents (ages twelve to ninteen). Alarmingly, obesity has quadrupled for children ages six to eleven. Because of these increases, obesity is now considered to be a public health crisis. The reason for concern is the fact that obesity contributes to, or makes worse, a number of illnesses. An obese person may suffer from one or more of the following:

- An overworked heart and circulatory system.
- Shortness of breath.
- High blood pressure.
- Diabetes.
- Poor capacity for physical activity.
- Strain on joints and ligaments resulting in pain.
- Poor adjustment to temperature change.
- Increased susceptibility to infectious disease.
- Psychological and social problems due to an obese appearance.

Most importantly, medical evidence shows that being overweight may shorten the span of life. For example, men who are 5 to 15 percent overweight are 44 percent more at risk of dying from circulatory conditions than men whose weight is what it ought to be.

The simple explanation for obesity has been overeating. A person was believed to become overweight by consistently eating more food than needed to maintain body tissues and provide for his or her basal metabolic rate and general level of physical activity. While basically true, this simple explanation does not provide an answer to the question of why some people eat to obesity while others do not.

Understanding the causes of obesity has been the goal of many researchers. By studying obesity, researchers have come to realize that obesity is a condition with not one, but many causes. The causes include genetic, biochemical, psychological, environmental, and cultural factors. These factors may operate individually or in relationship to one another.

Genetic studies have identified over 200 genes related to weight. Some researchers estimate that there may be as many as 1,000 genes that affect size and weight. Those who study brain-body chemistry have identified a number of hormones that influence obesity. Grhelin, an appetite stimulate, is one such hormone.

Grhelin is produced in the cells of the stomach and in the small intestine. When a person diets, the body feels threatened by starvation. To promote survival, the stomach increases the production of grhelin to stimulate appetite and encourage eating.

To date, the results of these, and other, genetic and biochemical studies have been promising enough for researchers to maintain that a number of genes and body chemicals contribute to obesity. Genes and hormones are believed to regulate such weight-related factors as appetite, food preferences, energy output, the number of fat cells in the body, the storage of fat in the fat cells, body weight set-point, and metabolism.

It is impossible to overestimate the importance of genetic and hormonal research in answering the question of why some people are obese. It should be very comforting to individuals who struggle with obesity to know that, in many ways, their obesity is not their fault. Their genes and hormones have been working against them because, in the words of researchers Peter J. Brown and Vicki K. Bentley-Condit in *The Handbook of Obesity*, "from the point of view of the body, there is no difference between purposeful dieting and unintended famine." (page 146) The research findings also give healthcare providers information important to the development of appropriate treatments for obesity, such as weight loss surgery.

In addition to these genetic causes, there are a number of psychological and social contributors to obesity. These psychological and social contributors may not cause obesity, but they may make a difficult situation worse. Common psychological factors that may contribute to overeating to severe obesity are depression, low self-esteem, social anxiety, and poor stress management coping skills.

Members of the bariatric and psychological communities have noted that a significantly high number of women who are severely obese have been a victim of abuse. The most frequent form is childhood sexual abuse. Neglect, poverty, parental mental illness, multiple step-parents or care takers, parental alcoholism or drug use, as well as physical battering, rape, and emotional abuse have also been reported. Individuals may eat in response to these abusive experiences to soothe themselves, or stuff down frightening feelings.

Social relationships and activities may play a very significant role in contributing to severe obesity. Families, friends, social and business groups may get together with eating the primary activity planned. Individuals may be encouraged to eat as a sign of being part of the group. In some instances, eating large quantities of food or conforming to a particular body size may be a requirement for being part of the group. In many families and marriages, conflicts over control and autonomy may take place around food and body size.

Whatever the contributing causes may be, severe obesity is a significant problem that hurts individuals, couples, and families. In 1993, writer Leslie Lampert dressed in a special-effects suit to add one hundred fifty pounds to her five-foot, six-inch frame. She had just watched the movie *Death Becomes Her* starring Goldie Hawn and Meryl Streep. In the course of the movie plot, Goldie eats to severe obesity. She wears a special-effects suit to add two hundred pounds to her frame. The film led Lampert to wonder what it would be like to be so big; what life would be like as an obese person. She designed an experiment in which she would live as an obese person for one week.

Each morning of the experiment, Lampert slipped into a "fat suit" custom-made by Richard Tautkus, a special-effects artist. Her life changed dramatically. In an article for the May, 1993, issue of Ladies Home Journal, Lampert wrote:

> *"One morning I gained one hundred fifty pounds, and my whole life changed. My husband looked at me differently, my kids were embarrassed, friends felt sorry for me, and strangers were shamelessly disgusted by my presence. The pleasures of shopping, family outings and going to parties turned into wrenchingly painful experiences. In truth, I became depressed*

by just the thought of running even the most basic errands…
But mostly, I became angry. Angry because what I experienced…
was that our society not only hates fat people, it feels entitled
to participate in a prejudice that at many levels parallels rac-
ism and religious bigotry. And in a country that prides itself
on being sensitive to the handicapped and the homeless, the
obese continue to be the target of cultural abuse."

As Lampert experienced, spouses and children are often embarrassed by or ridiculed because of the obesity and may add to the hurt the obese person feels. Spouses may choose to attend social functions alone. They may argue with the obese partner to lose weight and may try to control the kind and amount of food eaten. Children may not want the obese parent to drop them off at school or other activities in an attempt to avoid being teased by their peers. Even when family members are accepting of the obesity, the obese individual may feel so badly about their weight that they will not participate in the social activities of the family. Social isolation for protection becomes more important than disappointing their spouse or children.

At the end of her journalistic experiment, Leslie Lampert stepped out of her "fat suit" and returned to her life as an average weight person. Unfortunately, the genuinely obese cannot do the same. Instead, they have to try to find a way to cope with and function in a society that worships slimness and reacts to the obese individual with fear or hostility.

Some severely obese individuals have chosen to make peace with their obesity. Through psychotherapy, support groups, social clubs, and magazines such as Big and Beautiful, they have come to believe and proclaim that obesity is just a variation in size. It is not a sign that they cannot control themselves, that they are lazy, ugly, stupid, failures in life. And that is true. Obesity is not an issue of character, intelligence, or competence.

For other obese individuals, acceptance of their weight is not simple or sufficient. The physical, psychological, social, and economic issues are significant enough for them to pursue a more average body weight. To this end, they enroll in one weight loss program after another.

Traditionally, medical treatment for severe obesity has focused upon decreasing calorie intake and increasing physical activity. Commercial weight loss programs, as well as fad diets, have used the same formula. A seemingly endless number of liquid diets, pills, shots, foods, food supplements and exercise videos have been developed and promoted. Most claim to be the pathway to successful weight loss. Recognizing the psychological and interpersonal issues involved in being overweight, some medical and commercial weight loss programs include personal counselors and support or behavior modification groups for participants.

As discussed earlier, many people do lose weight as long as they remain on the selected low-calorie diet program and/or engage in exercise. But low-calorie diets are depriving. Even with support groups and behavior modification, few participants can stay on a depriving dietary program for very long. They are simply impossible to maintain. For many people, the on-going expense of a medical or commercial diet program becomes prohibitive. Due to frustration with the deprivation, a rate of weight loss that seems too slow, response to interpersonal pressure, or lack of money, a diet program is ended. The dieter usually returns to the prediet eating and physical activity level. Calorie consumption increases and the pounds pile back on, plus more.

It is estimated that 34% of adults in the United States are obese. If you are one of them, you have probably dieted many, many times in your life. You may have been successful only to regain all the weight you had lost, plus more. You may also have found that the more you diet and regain, the harder it becomes to lose. You want and need an alternative to the constant cycle of weight loss and regain. Fortunately, bariatric medicine provides several viable surgical alternatives for you.

Bariatrics is the name given to the area of medicine that treats obesity. Bariatric physicians use supervised low calorie diets, such as Optifast and Medifast, and/or pharmacotherapy (a variety of diet medications) to treat obesity. Bariatric surgeons use surgical procedures as treatment options.

Surgeons were called upon to develop safe, lasting treatments for weight reduction for the obese because of the significant failure rate of supervised low calorie diets and diet medications. It had been noted that irreversible operations that removed segments of the stomach and small bowel as treatment for some types of cancer and other illnesses resulted in dramatic weight loss. Although the amount of weight loss occurring after these surgeries was often life threatening, it was determined that modification of these surgical techniques might help seriously overweight people achieve and maintain a healthier body weight. To understand how bariatric surgery procedures work to produce weight loss, it is helpful to know a little about how the digestive process works.

The mouth is the beginning of the digestive system (*See figure 1*). In the mouth solid foods are broken up in the process of chewing (mastication). The salivary glands contribute liquid and enzymes to the chewed food making it easy to swallow. Swallowed food passes into the esophagus. The esophagus is a muscular canal about nine to ten inches long that connects the mouth to the stomach. Muscular fibers throughout the length of the esophagus propel food and liquid to the stomach through the process of peristalsis.

The stomach is an expandable organ that is a small wrinkled bag when it is empty. When food passes from the esophagus into the stomach, the walls of the stomach stretch. The average stomach stretches to hold about 32 to 48 ounces of food. In the stomach, food is mixed with several digestive juices (including pepsin, rennin, and hydrochloric acid). No absorption of nutrients takes place in the stomach.

From the stomach, food passes into the small intestine (small bowel). The small intestine is divided into three portions: the *duodenum*, the *jejunum*, and the *ileum*. The entire length of the small bowel is approximately 22 feet; its internal walls are pleated, like the folds of an accordion and are lined with *microvilli*. In the small intestine, food is broken down by a number of digestive juices (some produced within the small intestine and others produced by the liver, gallbladder and pancreas). Nutrients in the food are absorbed in the small intestine for use by the body. Most absorption of carbohydrates, proteins, and fats takes place in the jejunum and the first portion of the ileum.

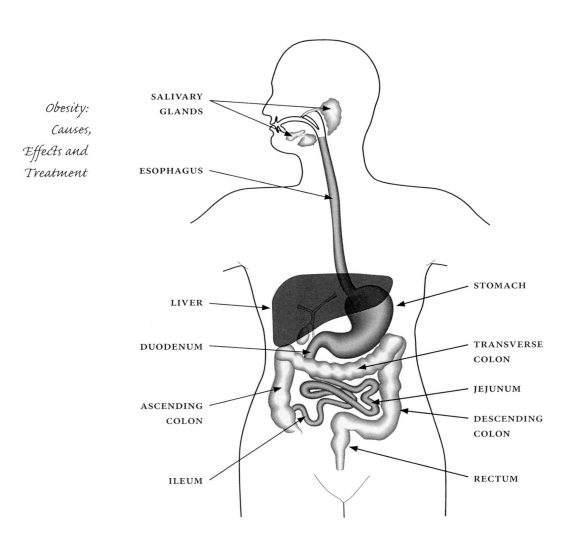

SALIVARY
GLANDS

ESOPHAGUS

LIVER

DUODENUM

ASCENDING
COLON

ILEUM

STOMACH

TRANSVERSE
COLON

JEJUNUM

DESCENDING
COLON

RECTUM

Figure 1 – *An Overview of the Digestive System*

Large portions of the small intestine may be removed without greatly hampering the absorption of nutrients. Because certain elements are absorbed in only a single area of the small intestine (such as B12 in the lowermost portion of the ileum, iron primarily in the duodenum, and folic acid in the upper jejunum) surgical removal of these areas results in deficiency.

Once processed by the small bowel, the food residue passes into the large intestine. The large intestine (colon), can be viewed as a waste processor that prepares the food residue to be eliminated from the body.

With their knowledge of the digestive process, bariatric surgeons experimented with procedures designed to help obese patients lose weight and keep it off. Two types of surgical procedures were tried. One type of procedure was malabsorptive; the other type was restrictive. The malabsorptive procedures reduced the absorption of calories and nutrients in the food consumed. The restrictive procedures reduced the amount of food that could be consumed.

One of the earliest malabsorptive procedures was Intestinal Bypass. The surgery bypassed large portions of the small intestine resulting in a significant reduction in the calories and nutrients absorbed from the food consumed. Patients did lose weight, but they experienced many serious complications including malnutrition, electrolyte imbalance, and chronic diarrhea. Some complications were resolved with a reversal of the procedure. Other complications were not resolved even when the procedure was reversed.

Horizontal Gastroplasty was an early restrictive procedure. Horizontal Gastroplasty partitioned the stomach into a small upper pouch and a larger lower pouch with a tiny outlet between the two. The intent of the surgery was to produce satiety (the feeling of fullness and satisfaction) with a reduced amount of food and by delaying the emptying of the stomach. The operation was relatively simple and had few complications. Its long-term results, however, were disappointing. The upper pouch stretched and the opening between the pouches enlarged. Patients felt hungry and were able to increase the amount and frequency of consumption. As a consequence, they regained weight. In most instances, patients regained all, or even more, of the weight initially lost following the procedure.

Treatments for Obesity...

11

Because of the high number of complications experienced with Intestinal Bypass and the high failure rate of Horizontal Gastroplasty, surgeries for weight loss became unpopular with many physicians and patients. In spite of the disappointing results, dedicated surgeons continued their experimentation. Today, weight loss surgeries are no longer experimental. More than 140,000 weight loss surgeries are done each year. The operations that have been developed are relatively safe and are achieving considerable success Public awareness and response has dramatically increased since celebrities such as Roseanne Barr (SRGB, aka Fobi-Pouch), Carnie Wilson and Al Roker (RNYGB) shared their positive experiences with weight loss surgery.

Robert

I was a heavy kid. I remember having to buy husky sizes in the boys department or having to shop in the men's department. In high school I wore a pants with a size 42 waist. I was heckled and laughed at a lot and I could never get dates. I went to my high school prom alone. After high school I only got dates because I had a good job and bought the women in my life whatever they wanted. I continued to be a laughing stock wherever I went. I was miserable. I felt that God must have a very cruel sense of humor to make me so large boned and obese. Because I figured this was just the way life was meant to be for me I decided to make food the love of my life. I also turned to alcohol to help me ease the pain that I felt inside.

In 1996 an event occurred that started a domino effect that changed my life forever. I slipped off some icy stairs twisting and breaking my foot, as well as ripping tendons and ligaments. Though I returned to my job as a truck driver six weeks after the accident, I continued to have trouble with my foot. Finally in 1997 I had to have surgery. After the surgery the doctor told me that I would probably never walk normally. The only way I could help my foot was to lose weight. At the time I was 458 pounds.

On my way home from the doctor I bought all kinds of junk food and five cases of beer. At home, however, I saw a commercial about surgery to lose weight. I called the number of the program and waited anxiously to receive the video about it. At first I felt it was the easy, cheater's way out. Then, again, I was already a loser weighing as much as did and being as miserable as I was. I went in for an appointment and had surgery.

It's now 1999 and I have lost 200 pounds in 13 months. I don't feel like a cheater at all. I feel like a winner! There was some pain involved in the surgery, but it is nothing compared to the emotional pain I felt being fat. I love the feeling of going into a store and buying normal size clothes off the rack. I also like the fact that people look at me without laughing. If you are overweight and are considering the surgery, do it. You'll be on your way to a whole new life. ❧

CHAPTER TWO

Weight Loss Surgery as a Treatment for Obesity

As discussed in Chapter One, we now understand that there are many complex factors contributing to obesity. We also understand that weight loss surgeries are the most effective means currently available to treat it. There are three types of surgery for weight loss: *restrictive, combined restrictive and malabsorptive*, and *malabsorptive*.

RESTRICTIVE WEIGHT LOSS SURGERIES

Although they may be smaller or larger, the average stomach is about the size of a football and holds a quart to a quart and a half of food (32 to 48 ounces). Restrictive surgical procedures are designed to encourage weight loss by dramatically limiting the amount of food that can be eaten at one time. Because the limitation in consumption is permanent, it is possible for weight loss to also be permanent. Restrictive weight loss surgeries include Gastric Banding, Vertical Gastroplasties, and Sleeve Gastrectomy.

Gastric banding involves placing a collar of synthetic material around the upper end of the stomach. This creates a small upper pouch of about a 3 to 4 ounce capacity. A narrow passageway allows food to flow from the small upper pouch into the larger lower portion of the stomach. (*See figure 2*)

Adjustable bandings use a hollow silicone collar that is connected to a tube with an outlet (port) located under the skin on the upper abdomen. Adding or removing saline solution through the port makes the collar tighter or looser. Adding saline inflates the collar narrowing the passageway and slowing the flow of food into the lower stomach. Removing saline solution deflates the collar enlarging the passageway and allowing food to flow more freely into the lower stomach. Adjustments in the collar are made by inserting a needle into the access port and are done while the patient is under x-ray.

Vertical Banded Gastroplasty (VBG) and Silastic Ring Vertical Gastroplasty (SRVG) involve sectioning off a small stomach pouch from the larger stomach. During the procedure, a vertical section along the small curve of the upper portion of the stomach near the esophagus is separated from the larger stomach by several rows of surgical steel staples. In VBG a strip of plastic mesh is placed through the stomach wall at the bottom of the stapled pouch to reinforce it and to maintain its size and shape. (*See figure 3*) In SRVG the outlet of the stapled pouch is reinforced and maintained by a small silicone tube. (*See figure 3*) The stapled pouch may, or may not, be divided from the larger stomach. Immediately following surgery, the stapled pouch will hold approximately 1 or 2 ounces. Gradually, the stapled pouch stretches to a maximum capacity of about 4 to 8 ounces.

The newest restrictive surgery is the Sleeve Gastrectomy. In this procedure the surgeon removes the left side (up to 90% of the greater curvature) of the stomach. The remaining stomach is roughly the size and shape of a small banana. (*See figure 4*) For some patients Sleeve Gastrectomy is the only surgical procedure used to treat their obesity. For patients with a BMI greater than 60 and/or who have medical conditions or a body shape that makes other weight loss surgeries too risky or difficult, Sleeve Gastrectomy may be the first stage of a two-stage surgical process. When medically safe, the Sleeve Gastrectomy is converted to a Gastric Bypass or Biliopancreatic Diversion/Duodenal Switch.

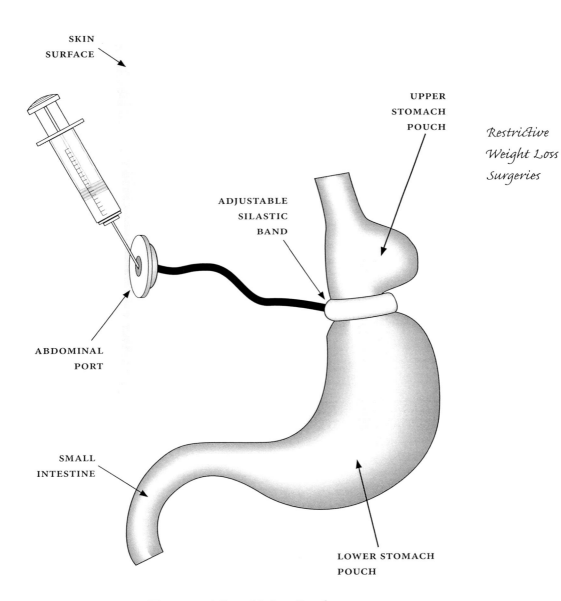

SKIN
SURFACE

UPPER
STOMACH
POUCH

*Restrictive
Weight Loss
Surgeries*

ADJUSTABLE
SILASTIC
BAND

ABDOMINAL
PORT

SMALL
INTESTINE

LOWER STOMACH
POUCH

Figure 2 – *Adjustable Lap-Band*

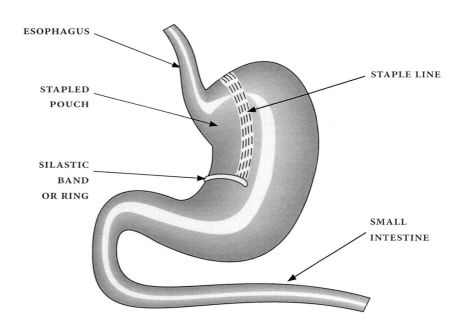

ESOPHAGUS

STAPLE LINE

STAPLED
POUCH

SILASTIC
BAND
OR RING

SMALL
INTESTINE

Figure 3 – *Silastic Ring Vertical Gastroplasty*

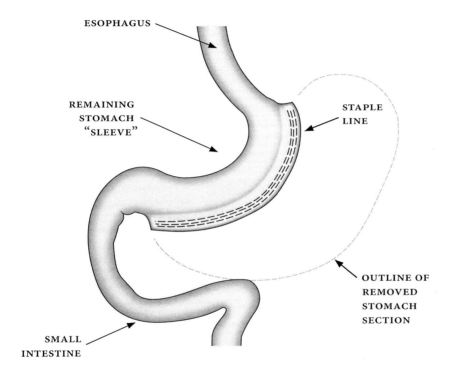

ESOPHAGUS

REMAINING STOMACH "SLEEVE"

STAPLE LINE

OUTLINE OF REMOVED STOMACH SECTION

SMALL INTESTINE

Figure 4 – *Sleeve Gastrectomy*

The restrictive surgeries help reduce weight only by limiting the amount of food that can be consumed at one time. Five-year follow-up studies suggest that restrictive surgeries, such as the Adjustable Lap-Band, VSG, and VBG, typically result in a weight loss of 47% of excess body weight. It is important to note that some patients lose more—or less—weight. The Sleeve Gastrectomy has not been done in the United States long enough to assess its long-term success but is likely to have a success rate similar to that of other restrictive surgeries. Regardless of procedure, to achieve the best possible weight loss, patients must follow a number of dietary and eating guidelines. These include the following:

- Eat the prescribed number of small meals per day.
- Do not snack between meals.
- Eat foods that are nutritious. Avoid "junk foods."
- Eat slowly and chew food to a pureed consistency before swallowing.
- Limit food intake to the recommended portion size or stop eating at the first sign of fullness.
- Avoid, or chew well, fibrous foods that may block the outlet to the lower stomach.
- Do not eat and drink fluids at the same time.
- Drink 64 ounces of low-calorie fluid per day.
- Vitamin and mineral supplementation may be necessary for some patients.

Inability to follow these guidelines may limit weight loss and/or lead to weight regain. Very poor dietary habits may lead to regaining even more than the pre-surgery weight. Patients who are unable to benefit from a restrictive surgery may choose to revise their procedure to one of the combined restrictive/malabsorptive or malabsorptive procedures.

The restrictive weight loss procedures do not alter the normal digestive process. As rapid weight loss may lead to the development of gallstones, a surgeon may recommend removal of the gallbladder at the time of surgery if preoperative tests reveal any sign of disease.

Restrictive procedures may be done by both the "open" and "laparoscopic" surgical methods and have a very low rate of possible surgical complication. In addition to the complications associated with any major surgery (to be discussed later) side effects of restrictive surgeries may include, but are not limited to, frequent vomiting, intolerance of some foods, constipation, blockage of the band or ring, poor emptying of the pouch due to constriction of the band or ring or to the build up of scar tissue, staple-line leak or failure (stapling procedures only), slippage of the band or penetration of the band into the stomach (lap-banding procedures only). Some—but not all—of the restrictive procedures are reversible. Reversal of a procedure typically leads to weight regain.

COMBINED RESTRICTIVE AND MALABSORPTIVE PROCEDURES

The combined restrictive and malabsorptive procedures maintain the creation of a small stomach pouch that reduces consumption capacity and adds a mildly to moderately malabsorptive component. To create the malabsorptive component the large lower portion of the stomach and a portion of the small intestine are bypassed delaying the mixing of food with gastric secretions and the bile and pancreatic juices needed to allow nutrients to be absorbed from the food consumed. There are three restrictive/malabsorptive procedures. These are the standard Roux-en-Y Gastric Bypass (RYGB/Proximal) the elongated Roux-en-Y Gastric Bypass (RYGB/Distal) and the Silastic Ring Gastric Bypass (SRGB).

The RYBG/Proximal has been the most common surgery done for weight loss in the United States. During the procedure, a small pouch at the top of the stomach just below the esophagus is stapled off completely. There is no exit to the lower portion of the stomach as with the purely restrictive procedures. The position of the pouch may be horizontal or vertical and it is typically divided (transected) from the large lower stomach. Although they may be shorter or longer, the length of the average small intestine is 22 feet. The small intestine is divided beyond the duodenum (a length of about 2 to 3 feet) and the longer portion of the intestine attached to the large intestine (the Roux limb, a length of about 19 to 20 feet) is attached to the stapled

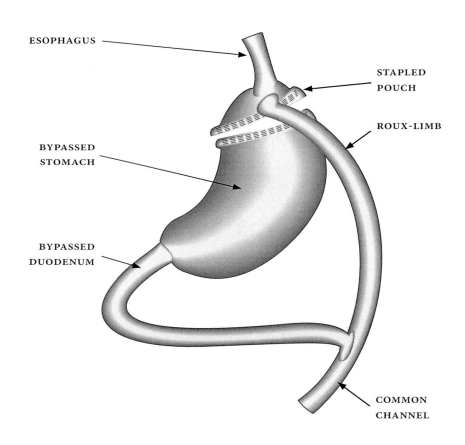

ESOPHAGUS

STAPLED
POUCH

ROUX-LIMB

BYPASSED
STOMACH

BYPASSED
DUODENUM

COMMON
CHANNEL

Figure 5 – *Proximal Roux-en-Y Gastric Bypass*

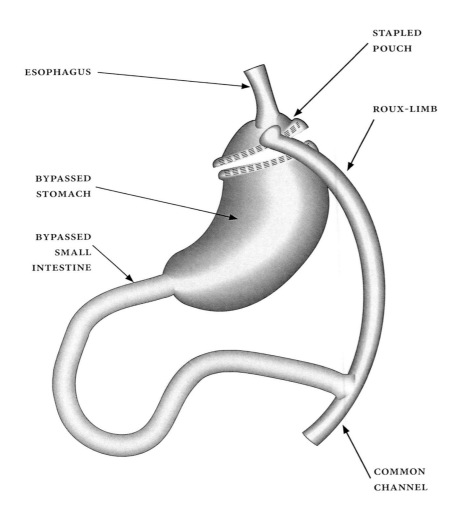

ESOPHAGUS

STAPLED
POUCH

ROUX-LIMB

BYPASSED
STOMACH

BYPASSED
SMALL
INTESTINE

COMMON
CHANNEL

*Combined
Restrictive and
Malabsorptive
Procedures*

Figure 6 – *Distal Roux-en-Y Gastric Bypass*

23

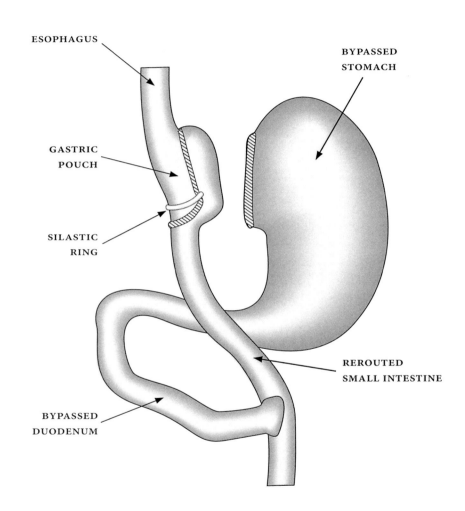

ESOPHAGUS

BYPASSED STOMACH

GASTRIC POUCH

SILASTIC RING

REROUTED SMALL INTESTINE

BYPASSED DUODENUM

Figure 7 – *Silastic Ring Gastric Bypass (SRGB) aka Fobi-Pouch*

pouch. The bypassed portion of the intestine is then reattached to the Roux limb creating a Y-shape. (*See figure 5*)

The RYGB/Distal is basically the same as the RYGB/Proximal procedure except for the length of the bypassed small intestine. In this procedure the length of bypass is approximately 6 feet instead of 3 feet. The longer bypass is designed to increase malabsorption encouraging greater weight loss and inhibiting weight regain. Because of the increased malabsorption, this procedure is sometimes classified as a malabsorptive procedure. As it mainly works by restricting consumption, it is included here in the combined restrictive/malabsorptive procedures. (*See figure 6*)

The SRGB (also known as the Fobi-Pouch) involves the creation of a stapled pouch of about 1 to 2 ounces. The very small size of the pouch is maintained by placing a silastic ring at the outlet between the pouch and the small intestine. The maintenance of the small size of the stapled pouch is designed to keep consumption very restricted in order to promote better weight loss and maintenance. The lower stomach and portion of small intestine are bypassed as in the RYGB/Proximal procedure. (*See figure 7*)

The consumption capacity of the RYGB/Proximal and Distal stapled pouch immediately after surgery is about 1 to 2 ounces. Over time, the stapled pouch does stretch to a consumption capacity of about 8 ounces. The size of the SRGB pouch is designed to be constant. As with the restrictive surgeries patients need to follow a special nutritional program that includes the following guidelines:

- Eat the prescribed number of small meals (typically 3 to 6) per day. Avoid snacking between meals.
- Eat foods that are nutritious and high in protein. Avoid junk food, especially high sugar foods.
- Eat slowly and chew food well before swallowing.
- Limit portion sizes to that recommended and/or stop eating at the first sign of fullness.
- Avoid drinking and eating at the same time.
- Drink 64 ounces of low-calorie fluid per day.

Inability to follow the dieting guidelines after surgery may result in weight regain. Vitamin and mineral supplementation is mandatory. Typically patients need to take a complete multivitamin daily. They may also need to take additional B1, B6, B12, as well as iron, calcium, and folic acid. RYGB/Distal patients may need additional A, D, E, and K. Failure to follow the nutritional guidelines may result in medical conditions associated with malnutrition.

Food tolerance is highly individual, but patients who have one of the combined restrictive/malabsorptive procedures can typically eat a wider range of foods than the purely restrictive surgery patients. The exception is the SRGB patients who may not tolerate fibrous food because of the ring. Two types of food intolerance are important to note for the combination restrictive/malabsorptive procedures. These are a possible intolerance of foods high in sugar and/or lactose.

When high sugar foods and beverages are rapidly consumed and released into the small intestine too quickly, the pancreas responds by overproducing insulin to lower the blood sugar. Sensations characterized by low blood sugar include lethargy, clamminess, shakiness and an overall feeling of weakness, rapid heartbeat, flushing of the skin, intestinal cramping and diarrhea. This is called "dumping." Anyone can experience the "dumping syndrome", but gastric bypass patients may experience it more frequently and severely because the re-routing of the intestine means that the release of foods and beverages into the intestine is no long regulated by the *pylorus* (the valve at the bottom of the stomach that gradually releases stomach contents into the intestine). In addition, the bypassing of a portion of the intestine allows sugary foods and beverages to reach the portion of the intestine that triggers the production of insulin more quickly.

There are two types of dumping: Early Dumping Syndrome (EDS) and Late Dumping Syndrome (LDS). Abdominal cramping and diarrhea are typical of EDS. LDS may include abdominal cramping and diarrhea but more typically includes sweating, palpitations, and weakness. Irritability of mood and behavior are also observed in both EDS and LDS. Clinical Dietitian Marie Genton researched the dumping syndrome and recommends that patients limit their intake of sugar to 15 grams or less in a 4-ounce serving of food or beverage to avoid dumping. Sally Myers, a Bariatric Dietitian, suggests that some patients may need to limit sugar intake to 3 grams or less. Many patients consider the possibility of dumping to be a positive component of the surgery because it limits the consumption of foods that may inhibit weight loss or contribute to weight regain.

Lactose intolerance is the inability to digest milk sugar (*lactose*). Lactase is an enzyme present in the portion of the small intestine called the proximal jejunum. Lactase breaks down lactose so that it can be absorbed into the blood stream. Lactose intolerance occurs in some patients because food does not come into contact with as much of this portion of the intestine and too little lactase is available to break down the lactose. This allows milk lactose to reach the colon without sufficient digestion. Symptoms of lactose intolerance include bloating, abdominal cramping, gas, diarrhea, and nausea. Using Lactaid milk and/or Lactaid tablets may reduce or resolve this problem. Some patients are advised to use soy, or other non-dairy products, instead of milk.

As with the restrictive surgeries, there are possible postsurgical complications. When done by a surgeon experienced in the procedures, the complications are low to relatively low in probability. In addition to complications associated with major surgery, possible complications for the combined restrictive/malabsorptive procedures include peritonitis (inflammation or infection in the abdominal cavity) following leakage from the stomach pouch or adjacent intestine and stoma (attachment of the small intestine to the stomach pouch), small bowel obstruction, malnutrition due to malabsorption, constipation, and hair loss. Because reduced digestion and malabsorption may affect absorption of medications, patients are advised not to take timed-release or enteric-coated pills. Adjustments in medication dosage may be necessary.

According to some five-year follow-up studies, combined restrictive/malabsorptive procedures typically result in a weight loss of 61.6% of excess body weight. As with all weight loss surgeries, patients do lose less or more weight depending on how diligently they follow post-surgical nutrition and exercise guidelines.

Restrictive/malabsorptive procedures do not require the removal of any organs, with the exception of the gallbladder if disease is evident. The pro-

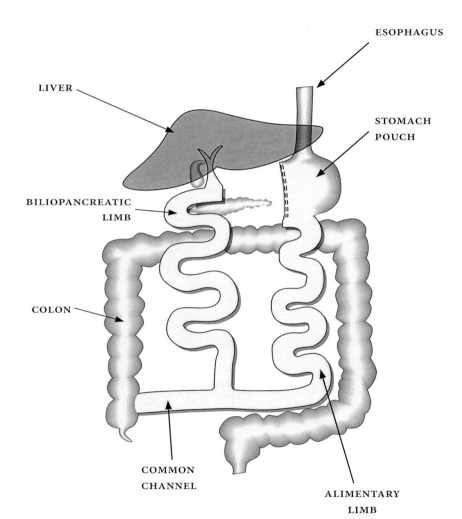

ESOPHAGUS

LIVER

STOMACH POUCH

BILIOPANCREATIC LIMB

COLON

COMMON CHANNEL

ALIMENTARY LIMB

Figure 8 – *Biliopancreatic Diversion* (BPD)

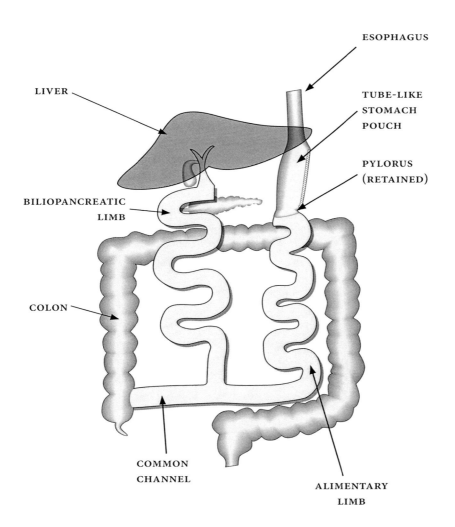

ESOPHAGUS

LIVER

TUBE-LIKE
STOMACH
POUCH

PYLORUS
(RETAINED)

BILIOPANCREATIC
LIMB

COLON

COMMON
CHANNEL

ALIMENTARY
LIMB

Figure 9 – *Biliopancratic Diversion/Duodenal Switch* (BPD/DS)

cedures may be done by either the open or laparoscopic methods. Although restrictive/malabsorptive procedures are not reversible (organs that have been partially removed cannot be replaced), they may be modified. Modification of the procedures typically results in weight regain. Patients who do not lose enough weight and/or who regain a significant amount of weight may choose to revise their surgery with one of the more malabsorptive procedures.

MALABSORPTIVE PROCEDURES

The malabsorptive weight loss surgeries are mildly restrictive and mainly malabsorptive. These procedures include the Biliopancreatic Diversion (BPD) and the Biliopancreatic Diversion/Duodenal Switch (BPD/DS). Extensive surgeries, the BPD and BPD/DS involve the removal of a portion of the stomach and a bypassing of a significant amount of the small intestine. The gallbladder and appendix are also removed in order to avoid possible confusion of symptoms of gallbladder disease or appendicitis with a complication of the procedure.

In the BPD the surgeon creates a smaller sized, rounded shaped, stomach by removing about three-fourths of the organ. The *pylorus* (the small valve at the bottom of the stomach, which regulates the release of stomach contents into the small intestine) is not retained. The small intestine is divided approximately in half and reconfigured into two channels. One channel is attached to the stomach and carries food. The other channel carries digestive juices from the liver and pancreas. The longer separation of food and digestive juices increases malabsorption (especially of fat) over that of the shorter gastric bypass procedures. The two channels of the intestine join together in a short common channel where a significant amount of nutrients in the food consumed is absorbed. (*See figure 8*)

The differences between the BPD and the BPD/DS are shaping of the new stomach into a tube rather than a ball, the retaining of the pylorus, and the manner in which the small intestine is divided and diverted. Surgeons who shape the stomach into a tube retaining the pylorus do so to prevent the dumping syndrome experienced by gastric bypass patients. There is, however, some question as to whether BPD patients do, in fact, experience dumping anyway.

In the BPD/DS the duodenum of the small intestine is left attached to the bottom of the stomach tube below the pylorus. The intestine is divided just below the place where the bile duct intersects with the intestine so that the drainage of the pancreatic juices and bile are bypassed. The remaining intestine is then divided approximately in half with the lower section reconnected to the duodenum. This lower portion of the intestine is called the alimentary channel and is attached to the large intestine or colon. The top portion of the divided intestine is reattached to the colon and becomes the common channel where food and digestive juices are combined for digestion. This is called the biliopancreatic limb. (*See figure 9*)

Although limited in portion size immediately after surgery, BPD and BPD/DS patients are often pleased that they can eventually eat average sized portions of food and experience little food intolerance. Patients do generally have a problem tolerating fat and experience diarrhea when they consume too much of it. The amount of fat that will cause diarrhea may vary from patient to patient. BPD and BPD/DS patients may also experience temporary or permanent lactose intolerance. It is important to note that the malabsorptive component does lead to permanent bowel change with patients having several small loose stools per day. Some patients do complain that their gas and stool has a foul odor.

Because the primary way these surgeries work to reduce weight is the malabsorption of calories and nutrients, eating a nutritious diet is essential. To protect health and achieve maximum weight loss, it is important to following these guidelines:

- Eat the number of meals recommended (typically 3 average to 6 small meals), by program guidelines. Do not snack between meals.
- Eat foods that are nutritious and high in protein. Avoid junk foods and high fat foods.
- Eat slowly and chew food well before swallowing.
- Limit portion sizes as recommended or stop eating at the first sign of fullness.

- Avoid eating and drinking at the same time or limit fluid consumption with meals.
- Drink 64 ounces of low-calorie fluid per day.

As with the combined restrictive/malabsorptive procedures, taking vitamin and mineral supplements daily is mandatory. Vitamins and minerals commonly recommended are a complete multivitamin, additional A, D, E, and K, B1, B6, B12, iron, calcium, and folic acid.

In addition to the complications typically associated with major surgery, possible side effects of the malabsorptive surgeries may include, but are not limited to, those of the combined restrictive/malabsorptive surgeries plus protein malnutrition, anemia, osteoporosis, and liver abnormalities. BPD/DS patients may be vulnerable to potassium deficiency.

Five-year follow-up studies suggest that the malabsorptive surgeries typically result in a weight loss of 70.1% of excess body weight with some patients losing less or more weight. The surgeries have a medium risk for possible surgical complications. Patients who experience malnutrition that cannot be managed with diet and supplementation often require revision of the surgery. Revision to one of the combination surgeries is necessary to discourage significant weight regain. BPD and BPD/DS patients, who cannot tolerate the foul gas and stool odor, sometimes have their surgery revised, as well. Malabsorptive surgeries are extensive and some surgeons think that they may not be safely performed by the laparoscopic method.

POSSIBLE RISKS AND COMPLICATIONS OF SURGERY

Major surgery has a number of possible risks and complications. For the weight loss surgery patient these may include, but are not limited to, allergic reaction to drugs, excessive bleeding, abscess, pneumonia, blood clotting, pulmonary embolism, cardiac arrhythmia, wound separation and/or infection, lung collapse, and hernia. Patient size and general health may influence surgical risks and complications, with those who are very large and/or who are in poor health being at increased risk. Therefore, it is important that only surgeons who are Board Certified and well experienced in treating obese patients perform weight loss surgeries.

Another important factor for possible risks and complications is patient compliance with post-surgical recovery guidelines. Patients must be a full partner with their surgeon in protecting their health. This means diligently following all treatment recommendations to the letter. Failure to do so increases risk and complication rates.

METHODS OF SURGERY

Traditionally, weight loss surgeries have been done via an "open" surgical method. The open method involves an incision down the midline of the torso from the breastbone to the navel or pubic area. The advantage of the open method is that it enables the surgeon to perform the procedure with a clear view and with "hands-on" precision.

Depending on the type of weight loss surgery done, and barring complications, hospitalization after an open procedure is typically 3 to 7 days. At home recovery is usually 4 to 6 weeks. Patients who have physically active jobs and are required to return to work without restriction may require a longer recovery period.

The severity, risks, complications, discomfort, scaring, and lengthy recovery time associated with the open method discourages some patients from having weight loss surgery. The application of the laparoscopic method to weight loss surgeries has decreased or resolved many of these issues. The laparoscopic method is less invasive, has fewer risks and complications, minimal discomfort and scaring, and a brief recovery time.

In the laparoscopic method, the surgery is performed with the aid of a fiber optic tube and light source attached to a small video camera. This instrument allows the surgeon to see the abdominal organs and manipulate the surgical instruments while viewing a TV monitor. The surgical instruments are inserted through several (4 to 6) small (¼ to ½ inch) incisions around the abdomen. The surgeon applies the same surgical principles of doing weight loss surgeries laparoscopically as would be done in an open procedure.

33

The laparoscopic method is not without risks. Therefore, it should be done by a surgeon who is not only experienced with weight loss surgery in general, but with laparoscopic weight loss surgery in particular. Depending on the type of surgery, and barring complications, hospitalization after a laparoscopic procedure is usually one to two days and at home recovery is a few days to a few weeks.

Not every weight loss surgery patient is a candidate for the laparoscopic method. Some surgeons may have size, shape, and distribution of fat requirements. Adhesions from previous abdominal surgeries or size and placement of organs may rule out the laporoscopic method. One of the most important goals for a surgeon is to complete surgery as safely as possible. Surgeons will advise patients before surgery about their appropriateness for the laparoscopic method and the possibility of needing to convert from a laparoscopic to an open method if it would be safer to do so.

CANDIDATES FOR WEIGHT LOSS SURGERY...

To qualify as a candidate for the surgical treatment of obesity most patients must meet a number of criteria. The most basic criteria used to determine candidacy is Body Mass Index or BMI. Surgical treatment for obesity is considered appropriate for patients with a BMI of at least 40 (roughly 100 pounds overweight) with no comorbid conditions and/or other risk factors or patients with a BMI of at least 35 (roughly 75 pounds overweight) with comorbid conditions and/or other risk factors. Comorbid conditions are medical conditions that are caused and/or made worse by obesity, such as hypertension, diabetes, sleep apnea, osteoarthritis, etc. The comorbidities would be expected to improve or be eliminated by significant weight loss.

In addition to meeting the BMI requirement, patients must have the mental or intellectual capacity to understand and comply with the recommended postoperative program. A patient must have a history of failing to lose weight or maintain weight loss on other diet programs. Candidates for bariatric surgery must not have any medical conditions that would make the surgical risks prohibitive or inappropriate, such as osteoporosis and/or cholelithiasis. A patient must demonstrate a willingness to engage in the lifestyle and nutritional habits known to support the achievement and maintenance of a healthy body weight. It is also advisable that patients have support from family, spouse, or close friends. Patients with psychological and interpersonal issues may be acceptable, especially if they are involved in psychotherapy.

Bariatric surgery is not recommended for the mentally ill or impaired, patients known to abuse alcohol and/or drugs, or those with an eating disorder such as *anorexia nervosa* or *bulimia nervosa*. Bariatric surgery is contraindicated for patients who are pregnant. Some surgeons have age restrictions.

PREOPERATIVE AND POSTOPERATIVE TREATMENT...

Individuals who select a weight loss surgery to achieve a healthy body weight are advised to consider carefully the selection of a surgical program. The bariatric community recommends that patients select a multidisciplinary program that provides preoperative education and assessment and postoperative follow-up and/or have qualified as a "Center of Excellence". Centers of Excellence are programs that have completed a rigorous certification process that assures they meet specific standards of multidisciplinary care.

Before surgery, a patient should explore with the surgeon all of the advantages and disadvantages of weight loss surgery. The patient's individual medical history, condition and expectations for the outcome of surgery should be discussed. A complete medical, nutritional, and psychosocial evaluation should be completed. These steps assist the surgeon to determine that there are no contraindications for surgery. This is especially important since obese patients may be at a higher risk for surgical complications. These steps also assist the multidisciplinary team members to assess the nutritional and lifestyle changes the patient may need to make following surgery.

Following surgery, the patient should anticipate regular appointments with the surgeon or an internist experienced with weight loss surgery who will follow their progress. The appropriate postoperative medical tests should be done, as needed, to insure the patient's health.

For maximum weight loss, support groups, behavior modification programs, and/or educational materials should be available. Individual consultation with a mental health professional, dietitian, and physical therapist familiar with the special needs of weight loss surgery patients should also be available. Some programs provide the services of a patient coordinator to assist and monitor the progress of patients and to provide them with access or referral to multidisciplinary professionals as needed.

Is a preoperative and postoperative program really important? A preoperative program is necessary to make sure that both the patient and surgeon have all the information necessary to make an intelligent and informed decision about the viability of surgery. Preoperative education lets the patient know what to expect before, during, and after surgery. The education also informs the patient of the life-long nutritional and lifestyle changes that are necessary or may occur following surgery.

For all but a very few patients, a postoperative behavior modification or support program has been found to be important to successful weight loss and for limiting the possible regaining of weight. In a study of VSG patients, James and William Shamblin observed that if patients missed follow-up in the first year after surgery, they lost significantly less weight (as much as 20% less) than those who did participate in follow-up. Those patients who participated in support or behavior modification training on a regular basis for one year or longer experienced the most weight loss with the least regaining of weight. The psychosocial interview helps identify patients who may need to participate in individual or group psychotherapy in addition to any behavior modification or support groups provided by a program.

Tani

I was an overweight child that had become an overweight adult. Already in my 30's I had high blood pressure, joint pain, bruised heels with heel spurs, shortness of breath, reflux problems, back problems, and swollen feet and ankles. Tying my shoes was exhausting. Forget sitting in movie theater seats or chairs with arms. I felt like a stuffed sausage. When I'd lie down at night, my chest felt like it was crushing my neck. I also had sleep apnea. I was afraid that one day I wouldn't wake up and my mother would find me dead. In spite of being overweight and all of the medical problems it caused me, food was my only source of pleasure.

At 325 pounds I often felt like the invisible woman. Funny how salespeople do not want to help an obese person. Other times I felt all too visible. People would gawk at me and just roll their eyes. I felt so undeserving because of my immense weight that I would allow people to verbally abuse me. I don't know how many times I heard, "Oh, you have such a pretty face. Have you ever tried dieting? Why don't you just try some self-control?" I smiled on the outside but I was crying on the inside. The truth is I had tried every new diet on the market. I read books, took diet pills, drank liquid diets, had shots, and participated in many local diet programs. None would work for me.

Then hope entered my life. In fact, I was given a chance at a completely new life. I had gastric bypass surgery. With the

I've been there...

help of my surgeon and his wonderful staff, I learned that I wasn't failing at the diets, they were failing me. With the help of gastric bypass I have gone from a size 32 women's jeans to a size 8 petite jeans in just 14 months! I feel great and all my health problems are gone. Life is good! If anyone says that losing weight doesn't change your life, well they haven't had gastric bypass surgery or met me! ❧

CHAPTER THREE

Questions and Answers about Weight Loss Surgery

The decision to have weight loss surgery is a very personal one. It should be made thoughtfully after careful consideration of what the procedures are, how they work, and their long-term effects on your life. To make a thoughtful decision, it is important that you learn as much about the surgeries as you can.

A good way to learn about the procedures is to ask questions. Below are some of the frequently asked questions about weight loss surgery.

Q *How does weight loss surgery assist weight loss?*

A There are three ways that weight loss surgery assists weight loss. Surgeries such as the Adjustable Lap-Band, VBG, VSGB, and Sleeve Gastrectomy help people lose weight by significantly restricting the amount of food that can be eaten at one time. Surgeries such as RYGB (Proximal and Distal) and SRGB (Fobi-Pouch) help people lose weight by significantly restricting the amount of food that can be eaten at one time and causing mild malabsorption of the calories in the foods that are eaten. Surgeries such as BPD and BPD/DS help people lose weight by slightly restricting the amount of food that can be eaten and causing significant malabsorption of the calories in the foods that are eaten.

Q *What causes the restriction in the amount of food that can be eaten?*

A In the Adjustable Lap-Band procedure, the restriction is created by using a band to divide the stomach into a small upper pouch, and a larger lower pouch. In VBG and VSGB the restriction is created by using staples to separate a small stomach pouch from the larger stomach. The restriction allows patients to eat only a few ounces of food at a time. In the Sleeve Gastrectomy, stomach size and capacity are reduced by removal of up to 90% of the organ.

Q *What does malabsorption mean?*

A *Mosby's Pocket Dictionary of Medicine, Nursing, and Allied Health, Third Edition*, defines malabsorption as the "impaired absorption of nutrients from the gastrointestinal tract."

Q *How does malabsorption occur following weight loss surgery?*

A Malabsorption occurs following one of the malabsorptive procedures for two reasons. First, the re-routing of a portion of the small intestine separates the digestive juices from the food that is eaten. Food cannot be digested and calories and nutrients cannot be absorbed without it being mixed with the digestive juices. Second, the "common channel" or length of intestine where food and the digestive juices do mix together is shortened so that less small intestine is available to absorb calories and nutrients. The more malabsorptive procedures (BPD and BPD/DS) have the longest separation of food and digestive juices and the shortest common channel where they are mixed.

Q *Who is a candidate for weight loss surgery?*

A To qualify as a candidate for weight loss surgery a patient must have a BMI of at least 40. In some cases, a patient may qualify as a candidate with a slightly lesser BMI of 35 if they have medical conditions that may be corrected or improved with weight loss. In addition to the weight requirements, a patient must have repeatedly failed to lose weight or maintain weight loss through traditional dieting methods. A patient must also have the mental or intellectual capacity to consent to surgery, to understand the recommended postoperative lifestyle requirements, and to comply with them.

Q *How do I decide which procedure is best for me?*

A The decision about which procedure is best for a given patient is made in consultation with a surgeon who specializes in weight loss surgery and understands the special medical needs of the obese patient. Factors important in the decision include existing medical condition, dietary patterns, and the ability of the patient to make the lifestyle changes needed for successful weight loss and maintenance following surgery.

The following guidelines may also be useful: 1) The less weight a patient needs to lose and the more disciplined they are in their dietary habits, the less surgery may be required to help them achieve a healthier body weight; 2) The more weight a patient needs to lose and the less disciplined they are in their dietary habits, the more surgery may be required to help them achieve a healthier body weight.

Q *How do I find a weight loss surgeon or program?*

A Your personal physician may be able to refer you to a weight loss surgeon or program. Some patients are referred "word of mouth" by family or friends who have had weight loss surgery or who know of someone who has. Also, many programs advertise on the Internet, in local newspapers, or on local television and radio stations.

Q *How do I select a surgeon?*

A It is important to select a surgeon who is Board Certified. This means that the surgeon has fulfilled all educational, residency, and other specialty qualifications required for practice. The surgeon should also be experienced in doing weight loss surgery and knowledgeable about the special treatment needs of obese patients. It is also helpful to select a surgeon

41

or program that provides a comprehensive presurgical and postsurgical educational and/or support program.

Q *Is weight loss surgery covered by medical insurance plans?*

A Many medical insurance plans do cover weight loss surgery. Some plans limit the types of weight loss surgical procedures covered. A patient must check their individual policy to see if the surgical treatment for obesity is a covered benefit. Often a weight loss surgeon or program will help the patient determine their benefits.

Q *If my insurance plan does not cover weight loss surgery at all, or the procedure that I want, what are my options?*

A Many employers provide a choice of medical insurance plans and allow employees to change plans as their medical needs change. If your medical insurance plan does not cover weight loss surgery or the procedure you want, check to see what plan options are available to you. If medical insurance coverage is not available, you may discuss the costs of financing the procedure with your surgeon or program.

Q *Are there any medical or psychological conditions that would keep someone from being able to have weight loss surgery?*

A Weight loss surgery is major surgery and there are always risks involved. Some medical conditions make may make it unsafe for a patient to have weight loss surgery. Your physician or weight loss surgeon can inform you of these conditions. Psychologically, a patient must be mentally and emotionally competent enough to understand what weight loss surgery is and to comply with the postoperative recovery and lifestyle changes necessary to support weight loss. In addition, they should not engage in substance abuse (*i.e.* alcohol and/or drugs) or an eating disorder (*i.e. bulimia nervosa*).

Q *Is preoperative medical testing necessary?*

A Preoperative medical testing is important for the safety of the patient. Testing may identify medical conditions unknown to the patient that require preoperative and/or postoperative treatment or may affect the viability of surgery.

Q *Is preoperative psychological consultation necessary?*

A Surgeons and programs that understand the lifestyle and psychosocial adjustments necessary for successful weight loss following weight loss surgery do include psychological consultation. The consultation should alert the patient and his/her treatment team members to any special behavior or lifestyle challenges the patient may experience following surgery. Some psychological conditions or behaviors may influence the viability or timing of surgery (*i.e.* Major Depression with Suicidal Ideation).

Q *There is a lot of conflicting information about weight loss surgery. Some say all surgical procedures are dangerous and lead to horrible complications. What is the truth?*

A It is true that some weight loss surgical procedures done in the past often led to serious, life-threatening complications. These procedures are no longer done. The newer weight loss surgeries have been designed to promote weight loss with fewer possible complications. Three of the procedures, the Adjustable Lap-Band, Vertical Stapled Gastroplasty (vsg), and Roux-en-Y Gastric Bypass (rnygb) have been approved by the National Institutes of Health as relatively safe and reliable treatments for obesity.

   In addition to having the procedure done by a Board Certified surgeon experienced in doing weight loss surgery, patients must comply with postoperative treatment recommendations. Many common complications are a result of a patient's failure to follow the recommended postoperative recovery and lifestyle behaviors. If the recommended behaviors are followed carefully, many possible complications can be avoided.

Q *How much food can I eat after weight loss surgery?*

A The amount of food that can be eaten depends on the type of weight loss surgery a patient has had. Immediately after surgery, all of the procedures allow a very small amount of food to be consumed, perhaps as little as one or two ounces. The restrictive procedures allow a patient to eat only a few ounces at a time (typically less than a cup) for life. The combined procedures may allow patients to eat about a cup of food at a time. The malabsorptive procedures may allow patients to eat small to average size

43

portions of food. The exact amount of food that can be eaten will depend on the actual size of a patient's stomach pouch after surgery, the consistency of the food consumed, how carefully the food is chewed, and how quickly the food passes from the stomach pouch into the intestine.

Q *Do calories have to be counted after surgery?*

A Some patients mistakenly believe that weight loss surgery will help them lose weight without their having to be concerned about calorie intake. Calories do count after weight loss surgery. For successful weight loss, most surgeons or programs give calorie intake guidelines to their patients. Eating more calories than recommended may result in a plateau and/or contribute to weight regain.

Q *Isn't a patient hungry eating so little food and so few calories?*

A Hunger is a complex biological, biochemical, and psychological experience. True hunger is triggered by the nutritional needs of the body and/or by the feeling of emptiness in the stomach. Patients typically feel satisfied eating a small amount of food at a time. They do not feel the hunger associated with traditional dieting. Like average weight people, patients will get hungry every 3 to 5 hours.

Q *What if a patient does feel hungry?*

A The feeling of hunger can indicate several things. During the time the stomach is healing from surgery, a patient's dietary program usually consists of several small meals. Foods consumed are usually liquid or pureed in form. As the stomach heals, foods of a more solid consistency are added to the diet. Hunger may indicate that the stomach is healing and ready for an increase in the volume or consistency of foods consumed. Patients are asked to check with their surgeon and/or program dietitian before changing the amount or types of foods eaten.

Hunger may also have two other causes. First, a patient may be spacing meals too far apart. If so, the patient may need to eat more frequently. Second, a patient may be eating foods that empty too quickly from the pouch. If this is the case, a patient should eat foods that are high in nutri-

44

tion and take time to empty from the pouch. Eating foods that are high in fat or sugar and/or that empty from the pouch quickly usually leads to the feeling of hunger.

Q *Can a patient be healthy eating so little food and so few calories?*

A The health of the patient should be the primary concern of any weight loss surgery program. A patient can be healthy when eating a low-volume, low-calorie diet if the diet is carefully planned to meet the nutritional needs of the body. A good weight loss surgery program will include a professional (dietitian, nurse) who can provide dietary guidelines to patients. Taking vitamins is mandatory following many weight loss surgery procedures.

Q *How does a patient stop losing weight once they reach their goal weight?*

A Many patients find that they reach a satisfactory, natural plateau at or above their goal weight. If this happens, the patient simply continues following their current dietary program. If a patient begins to lose too much weight, their dietary program must be adjusted. Typically, the number of calories consumed at each meal is increased or the patient is told to add a small additional meal to their dietary program. It is important not to add too many calories or snack between meals. To do so may cause weight regain.

Q *What are the recommended recovery and lifestyle behaviors for successful weight loss?*

A Following surgery, patients are placed on a special dietary program to allow the stomach to heal from the surgical procedure. Because of the small size of the pouch, patients usually need to change the way they eat. They will need to eat small bites of food, chew the food to a pureed consistency, and eat very slowly. A life-long lifestyle of good nutrition and exercise is also important. Some patients need to change unhealthy or sabotaging attitudes, activities, and behaviors.

Q *How much weight can a patient expect to lose after weight loss surgery?*

A The exact amount of weight a person can lose after surgery depends on two variables. The first variable is the type of surgery. Some five-year follow-up studies suggest that patients lose less weight with the restrictive procedures, more weight with the combined restrictive-malabsorptive procedures, and even more weight with the malabsorptive procedures (typically 47%, 61.6% and 70.1% of excess body weight respectively). The second variable is how many of the recommended lifestyle changes a patient makes after surgery. The more committed a patient is to following the dietary program, exercising, and developing attitudes and behaviors that help them cope with stress without eating, the more weight a patient can lose.

Q *How much weight must a patient lose to be considered successful?*
A Weight loss—even after weight loss surgery—is affected by many factors. These include genetics, medical conditions, medications, as well as eating behavior. Surgeons often strive to help patients lose about 50 percent of their excess body weight (a loss of about 20 to 25 percent of weight at the time of surgery). Studies suggest that 50 to 70 percent of all weight loss surgery patients achieve this goal—meaning 30 to 50 percent do not.

Rather than focus on weight loss as the sole measure of success, it is helpful to note several additional factors. For example, can the patient follow the healthy lifestyle guidelines with the help of surgery; has health improved and/or need for medication decreased; can the patient participate in life more fully? Additionally, do they feel more attractive, feel more socially at ease and/or experience increased opportunity in their job or career? If so, they may consider themselves successful.

Q *Why do some patients fail to lose weight or sustain weight loss after weight loss surgery?*
A While there can be medical conditions or surgical complications that contribute to failure, the most common reasons are behavioral. Patients fail to lose weight or sustain weight loss because they do not make the recommended lifestyle changes and follow them for life. This includes having a weight loss/weight maintaining dietary program and engaging in regular exercise. Eating foods too high in calories, snacking

46

between meals, and a sedentary lifestyle inhibit weight loss or result in weight regain.

Q *If patients have to watch their calories and exercise, why have weight loss surgery?*

A To maintain a healthy body weight, even average weight people must watch their calorie intake and/or exercise regularly. For the reasons described in Chapter Two, individuals who are obese have been unable to control their calorie intake. Exercise is often difficult or avoided because of pain caused by the excess weight. Weight loss surgeries permanently restrict the amount of food a patient can consume and/or reduces absorption of calories consumed. These factors make it possible for the obese patient to better control calorie intake. As they lose weight, exercise becomes more comfortable, and even enjoyable.

Q *How fast can a patient lose weight after weight loss surgery?*

A A number of factors influence rate of weight loss following surgery. These include the type of surgery a patient has had, the size of a patient at the time of surgery, and how carefully a patient follows post-surgical dietary guidelines. Patients who have had a restrictive or combined restrictive and malabsorptive procedure may lose 1 to 3 pounds per week. Those who have had a primarily malabsorptive procedure may lose more weight per week. All patients will experience an inconsistency in their rate of weight loss. Brief plateaus are also to be expected.

Q *Is loose skin to be expected after weight loss surgery?*

A The elasticity of the skin varies from patient to patient. Most patients who have one hundred pounds or more to lose will have some loose skin. Exercising to develop good muscle tone will help decrease the appearance of loose skin. Careful dressing helps to conceal it. Some patients elect to have cosmetic or corrective surgery to tighten the skin. It is recommended that cosmetic or corrective surgery be done only when a patient has lost as much weight as they can and/or has reached goal weight.

Q *How big is the incisional scar or scars?*

A. The size of the scar(s) depends upon the type and method of surgery done. Patients whose surgery is done laparoscopically will have several small incisional scars around the abdomen. Patients who have surgery done by the open method will have a long mid-line incision from the breastbone to the navel or pubic area. Surgeons can recommend treatments to help the incision(s) heal so that they are as "invisible" as they can possibly be.

Q *What possible surgical complications are sometimes associated with weight loss surgery?*

A Because weight loss surgery is major surgery, complications may include (but are not limited to) allergic reaction to drugs, organ perforation, blood clots, cardiac arrhythmia, pulmonary embolism, wound separation or infection, and gastric leak.

Q *What long-range complications are associated with weight loss surgery?*

A Complications for all bariatric surgery patients include (but are not limited to) hair loss, intolerance of some foods, malnutrition. Those who have had an open method procedure may develop hernia(s). Those who have had a restrictive or combined restrictive/malabsorptive procedure—especially one using a silastic ring or band—may experience ring obstruction and/or chronic vomiting. Procedures involving stapling with transection of the stomach pouch and rerouting of the small intestine may develop gastric leaks and peritonitis. Procedures involving rerouting of the small intestine may lead to bowel obstructions.

Q *What benefits may I expect after weight loss surgery?*

A There are many benefits that may be experienced with weight loss after surgery. The most important benefit is improved health. Patients are typically able to reduce or discontinue medication and experience reduced physical discomfort and pain. Patients are often able to breathe and move about more easily. Many patients also report improved self-esteem, self-confidence, and quality of life. Social, educational, and career opportunities are often enhanced.

Q How long is a patient in the hospital after weight loss surgery?

A Barring complications, the length of hospital stay depends on the type of procedure done, the method of surgery, and general health of the patient. Patients who have a laparoscopic restrictive or combined restrictive/malabsorptive procedure may go home within one to two days. Patients who have any procedure done by the open method may go home within three to seven days.

Q How long is a patient off work?

A As with length of hospital stay, time off of work depends on the method of surgery, the general health of the patient, and the type of work they do. A patient who is in good health, has a job that is not very physically demanding, and who has surgery laparoscopically often returns to work in a few days or few weeks. A patients who experiences poor health, has a physically active job, or who has surgery by the open method may be off work four to six weeks. A patient who has a physically demanding job and/or who cannot return to work with any performance restriction will need to be off as long as it takes to recover enough to do their job.

Q Are there any restrictions in physical activity following weight loss surgery?

A Once fully recovered from surgery, most patients find that their physical activity is less restricted than it was before surgery. There are no long-term restrictions in activity.

Q If internal staples are used in the surgery, will they set off the security alarm at an airport?

A No, they will not.

Q Should a patient tell people they are having or have had weight loss surgery?

A Disclosure of weight loss surgery is an individual decision. Some patients are very open and freely discuss their surgery. Others are more private and wish to keep it a secret from all but their closest family members and friends. It is best for patients to do what is most comfortable for them.

Q *Will surgery be painful?*

A The experience of pain varies between surgical methods. The laparo-scopic method is typically less painful than the open method. Pain also varies between patients. Those with a high pain tolerance usually experi-ence less discomfort than those with a low pain tolerance. Surgeons do not want patients to experience unnecessary pain. It is important that patients communicate with their surgeon and nursing team about their experience of pain. The treatment team will then do everything possible to minimize discomfort.

Q *Are the procedures ever reversed?*

A The procedures are designed to be permanent in order to encourage maxi-mum weight loss and maintenance. Some—but not all—procedures may be reversed or modified if medically necessary. For example, a restrictive procedure such as the Lap-Band may be reversed by removing the band or a combined restrictive/malabsorptive procedure such as the Gastric Bypass or a malabsorptive procedure such as the BPD/DS may be modified by lengthening the amount of intestine absorbing calories and nutrients. Weight regain typically occurs with reversal or modification.

Q *What happens to the big part of the stomach that is divided from the stomach pouch in the combined restrictive/malabsorptive procedures?*

A The big part of the stomach remains healthy; it just does not participate in the digestive process as it did before. Any digestive fluids secreted into the stomach pass into the intestine to participate in the digestive process.

Q *What about pregnancy after weight loss surgery?*

A Women do have babies after weight loss surgery. Physicians usually recom-mend that a woman not get pregnant for at least one year following surgery. As with any pregnancy, good prenatal care is essential. Patients will need to monitor their eating behavior to make sure that food choices provide adequate nourishment. Some patient's may require special nutritional supplementation. Patients may gain little weight during pregnancy.

Q *What can a patient expect emotionally following weight loss surgery?*

A For a short time after surgery, many patients report some irritability or depression. This is usually attributed to the normal recovery experience and food restrictions after surgery. As patients recover, adjust to their new dietary guidelines, and lose weight, these feelings are replaced by the excitement of success and feeling of being in control of their eating behavior. Some patients experience significant emotional distress if they were emotional, compulsive, or binge overeaters before surgery and can no longer engage in these behaviors. Emotional distress is also experienced if patients have unrealistic body or life expectations and/or difficult relationship adjustments after surgery.

Q *Are there and "forbidden foods" after weight loss surgery?*

A Programs vary on their post-surgical dietary guidelines. Some have "forbidden foods" and others allow eating most foods in moderation. Whatever the program food guidelines, it is important to follow them to the best of your ability.

Q *Are there some foods that can't be tolerated after weight loss surgery?*

A Food tolerance varies from surgery to surgery and patient to patient. Patients who have a restrictive surgery may eat almost everything they ate before surgery. They just have to eat more carefully and consume smaller portions. Some patients do find that they can no longer tolerate fibrous meats, doughy breads, and some raw fruits and vegetables. Patients who have had a combined restrictive/malabsorptive procedure also need to eat more carefully and consume smaller portions. They may also have difficulty eating fibrous meats, doughy breads, and some raw fruits and vegetables. The combined procedures may also make some patients sensitive to sugar. Eating or drinking foods high in sugar may result in "dumping." Patients who have a mostly malabsorptive procedure can eat almost any food. As they have difficulty digesting fats, they may experience diarrhea if they eat fatty foods. Lactose intolerance may be a side effect of surgery.

Q *What is "dumping" and how do patients know it is happening to them?*
A Dumping is associated with the rapid ingestion of large amounts of high carbohydrate foods and beverages, especially those high in sugar. Anyone can experience dumping but patients who have had a combined restrictive/malabsorptive procedure may experience it more frequently and severely because of the rerouting of the small intestine. The rerouting of the intestine means that the release of foods and beverages is no longer regulated by the pylorus (the valve that releases foods and beverages from the stomach into the intestine). In addition, the bypassing of the intestine means that sugary foods and beverages too quickly reach the portion of the intestine that regulates blood sugar. This causes the pancreas to overproduce insulin to lower the blood sugar. Sensations characteristic of low blood sugar include lethargy, clamminess, shakiness, an overall feeling of weakness, a rapid heartbeat, flushing of the skin, and/or diarrhea. Patients know they are dumping when some, or all, of these sensations occur.

Q *What is lactose intolerance and how do patients know it is happening to them?*
A Lactose intolerance is the inability to digest milk sugar (called lactose). Lactase is an enzyme present in the portion of the small intestine called the *proximal jejunum*. It breaks down the lactose so that it can be absorbed into the blood stream. Lactose intolerance occurs following the combined and more malabsorptive weight loss surgeries because food does not come into contact with this portion of the intestine and too little lactase is available to break down the lactose. This allows the milk lactose to reach the colon without sufficient digestion. In the colon, the milk lactose ferments and produces excess hydrogen. The excess hydrogen causes bloating, cramps, gas, diarrhea and nausea. Limiting the consumption of milk and milk products often successfully resolves this condition. Using Lactaid milk or Lactaid tablets may also be helpful.

Q *Does weight loss surgery affect relationships?*
A Significant weight loss following weight loss surgery may affect relationships. Good relationships often stay the same or get better. Stressed re-

lationships may stay the same or become more stressed. It is important to understand that as you change your lifestyle, the people close to you will be affected by the change. To support your weight loss, family members and friends may find it necessary to change some of their lifestyle behaviors, too. Some may be willing to do this while others are not.

Q *Why do vitamins and other pills need to be crushed or chewed following some weight loss surgeries?*

A The restrictive surgeries require everything that is consumed to fit through a very narrow opening or silastic ring. Large pieces of food or whole pills may block the opening or ring or just sit in the stomach pouch because they can't get through. To avoid possible blockage, it is recommended that vitamins and other pills be taken in a liquid form, chewed, or crushed. The stomach pouch created in the combined procedures is very small and the reattachment of the small intestine to the pouch is very narrow right after surgery. It is recommended that vitamins and pills be taken in a liquid form, chewed, or crushed for about four weeks. After that time, small pills may be swallowed one at a time. Large pills may still need to be crushed or chewed. A physician or pharmacist can answer questions about whether certain pills can be chewed or crushed without affecting the way they work within the body.

Q *Have any patients regretted having weight loss surgery?*

A There are some patients who have regretted having weight loss surgery. Those who do regret having it usually do so because of the social pressure from friends and/or family. Others dislike the lifestyle changes needed. Overwhelmingly, most patients are glad that they had a weight loss procedure. They feel that the benefits of surgery are far greater than the challenge of any lifestyle, emotional, and relationship adjustments they need to make.

The questions and answers above may not satisfy all of your concerns about weight loss surgery. Your surgeon and other program treatment team members can address additional questions for you. Patients who have had surgery may be good sources of information, too. Remember, no question is too silly or stupid. The more informed you are about weight loss surgery, the better able you will be to decide if, and what, particular weight loss surgery is right for you. The knowledge you gain will also prepare you to achieve your weight goal following a weight loss procedure.

Questions and Answers about Weight Loss Surgery

Part Two

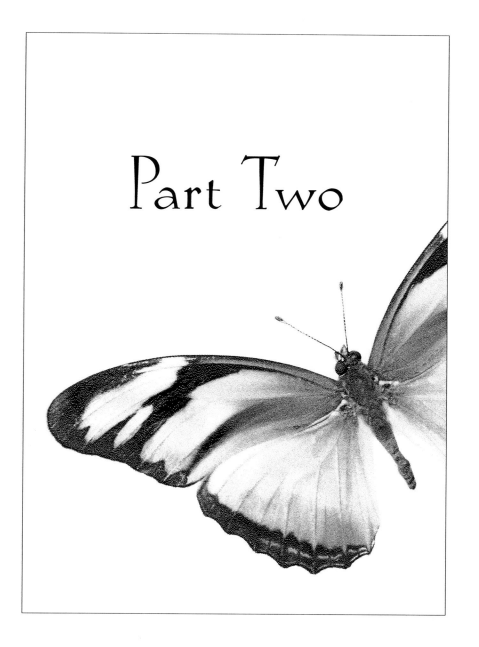

Breanna

For as long as I can remember, I have had a weight problem. As a child and teenager I kept it somewhat under control because I was very active in sports. After high school, with no sports to fall back on, I really started to put the pounds on. I never replaced my sports activities with another exercise program. This proved to be my downfall. As the years went by, my weight increased more and more. I tried a variety of diets on and off well into my thirties. Each diet left me in even worse shape than the one before.

One day I was pursuing my favorite activities... watching TV and eating. On TV I saw a commercial for a weight loss program that promised permanent weight loss. I though it was just another one of those "get your money" schemes aimed at me and other desperate obese people.

Because I was desperate, I called anyway. Shortly after my call to the 800 number, I was sent information about the procedure of gastroplasty and given the number of the program coordinator in my area. It took a while, but one day I did call. The coordinator told me all about the program and that gastroplasty was major surgery. After hearing all about the procedure and the program, I felt that it was the help I needed.

My excitement about finding an answer quickly turned to disappointment. I found out my insurance provider , an HMO, did not cover the procedure. A year went by and I needed to change insurance companies. I was hopeful that my new insur-

ance company would cover the surgery. I called my program coordinator and she did some checking for me. She found out that this insurance provider did not cover the surgery either. By this time a second surgery had become available. This surgery was gastric bypass. Gastric bypass was explained to be a gastroplasty with a rerouting of the small intestine. The rerouting of the small intestine made it difficult to eat foods high in fat and/or sugar. Because of my life-long habit of eating high fat foods, I knew gastric bypass was the right surgery for me. I changed insurance companies again.

By this time my problems had become worse. I had injured my back and been off work for six months. To recover from my back injury, I had to be even less active than I already was (if that was possible). My weight ballooned to 350 pounds… the highest it had ever been. I was very unhappy and painfully miserable. My orthopedic surgeon told me that until I lost weight, my back problem was only going to get worse. He asked if there was anyway he could make things better for me. I told him about my desire to have gastric bypass to help me permanently lose weight. He agreed to write a letter to my insurance provider explaining my medical condition and how gastric bypass would help me.

With the help of my orthopedic surgeon, my program coordinator, and a wonderful lady at my third insurance company, I was finally approved for surgery. I am so thankful to these people for all their help. I had gastric bypass on April 8, 1994. At this time I am about 80 pounds from my goal weight of 150 pounds!

Having gastric bypass has not only helped with my weight problem, it has helped my life in so many other ways, too. I have found new friends for life and my back, though not healed, is better. Also, to keep me from sitting at home and going absolutely crazy, I have become a volunteer in my program. Is that great or what? I am so grateful I have had gastric bypass and have so many wonderful new friends and opportunities in my life! ❧

CHAPTER FOUR

Living Comfortably with your Surgical Tool

Part One of this guide began with something you already know. Diets don't work for most people—especially the severely obese. Most dieters find themselves in the dieting "yo-yo" syndrome. They lose weight only to regain it again and again and again, plus more.

Fortunately, for the severely obese there are alternatives to the lose weight regain it cycle. Weight loss surgery procedures have been found to be effective tools for weight loss. They help up to 85 percent of those who have the procedures achieve and maintain a healthier body weight.

The most important word to remember is "tool." Weight loss surgeries are not magic, they are just tools. To paraphrase a song Helen Reddy made popular, they are strong, but not invincible. Like any tool, it must be well cared for if it is to last. The tool must also be used properly if it is to provide maximum results.

Some may ask, "If the procedures are just tools, why have them done at all? What is the benefit?" The benefit is that weight loss surgery significantly

59

increases the chances of losing weight and keeping it off permanently. While dieting has a success rate of 5 to 20% (perhaps just 1% for the obese), weight loss surgery has a success rate of 47 to 70.1% (some patients do lose less or more). Who would not want to benefit by such a tremendous increase in the odds for success!

The study reported earlier by James and Richard Shamblin was conducted on three thousand nine hundred gastroplasty patients. The research indicated that 90 percent of the group lost at least 40 percent of their excess weight. The only variable in terms of how much excess weight they lost was how diligently they followed the postoperative lifestyle recommendations. While weight is lost following weight loss surgery, how much weight is lost will depend on how earnestly the lifestyle habits that promote successful weight loss and maintenance are followed. What are those lifestyle habits?

Dr. Judith Stern, professor of nutrition and internal medicine at the University of California at Davis, was very interested in learning about when diets work and when they don't. On the one hand were women who repeatedly lost weight only to regain it. On the other hand were women who lost weight and kept it off.

To understand what made some women succeed while others did not, Stern and two colleagues questioned close to fifteen hundred women. They talked to a control group who never had a weight problem, a maintainers group who had lost up to 20 percent of their excess weight and kept it off for two years, and a regainers group who lost some weight but put it back on again. What Dr. Stern and her colleagues found was that those who lost weight and maintained it replaced weight-gaining behaviors with weight-losing habits. Practiced faithfully, these habits have become a new and permanent way of living which enables them to maintain a healthier weight.

Maintainers have learned to do the following:
1. Give up dieting… forever! Instead of dieting, maintainers practice a healthy way of eating based on the nutritional needs of their bodies.
2. Stop being a couch potato! Maintainers engage in regular physical exercise to burn fat and increase the metabolism.

3. Don't go it alone! Maintainers get help from spouse or companion, family and friends, a support group, or psychotherapist.
4. Stop being dishonest! Maintainers look honestly at their self-sabotaging attitudes and behaviors. They develop positive attitudes and behaviors that support their weight loss.
5. Stop reacting to stress! Maintainers realize they turn to food to cope with problems. They practice proactive stress management, problem solving, and relaxation techniques.

All of these habits are important to weight loss surgery patients if they are to lose as much of their excess weight as is possible or if they are to avoid regaining some of the weight lost. In addition to these, one more lifestyle habit is important following the surgery. This is to care for and protect the stapled pouch.

In this chapter, and in the remainder of Part Two, all of these lifestyle habits will be fully discussed with special consideration of the weight loss patient. The first lifestyle habit for consideration is that necessary to protect the stapled pouch.

CARING FOR THE HEALING WEIGHT LOSS SURGICAL PROCEDURE...

Weight loss surgery programs often have special dietary guidelines for patients to follow for a few days or weeks after surgery. These guidelines include a meal schedule, a list of what types of foods that may be consumed, and a description of the exact amount of each type of food that is to be consumed at each meal. These guidelines are designed to do four things:

1. Provide for the basic nutritional needs of the body.
2. Allow the anatomical changes in the body to heal securely (*i.e.* the transected stapled pouch and rerouted/reattached small intestine).
3. Encourage the gradual stretching of the stapled pouch from its minimum to its maximum capacity.
4. Promote tolerance of a variety of foods.

To promote comfort in eating and to protect the healing stomach and/or intestine, patients are advised to following these guidelines:

1. Eat slowly and carefully. Always chew small bites of food to a pureed consistency. Take twenty to forty minutes to eat a meal. Liquids are a good choice if there is only twenty minutes to eat. Eat more solid foods when there is adequate time to eat them slowly.
2. Stop food intake if any pain develops. Pain may develop if liquids are sipped or foods are eaten too quickly, or if too much is taken in at one time. The pain may be felt in the left shoulder and/or the esophagus. If pain develops, wait two hours, or until the pain subsides, to resume food intake.
3. Pay attention to how the stomach feels. Stop eating as soon as any sensation of fullness is experienced. The softer the food being eaten, the more of it may be consumed before fullness is felt.
4. Because some people cannot tell when they are getting full, it is best to limit recommended portion size to no more than eight ounces of food at a time.

The importance of following these guidelines cannot be over emphasized. Failure to follow them may lead to a number of negative consequences. At the very least, patients may experience discomfort and/or vomiting. At the very worst, they may experience leakage at the staple line or at the anastomoses (places where the intestines are reattached during surgery). Discomfort and/or vomiting, while uncomfortable, are not medical emergencies. Leakage is a medical emergency.

A number of weight loss surgery programs in Southern California use the five-phase nutritional program described below as a way of caring for the healing surgical procedure. It is given only as an example of a postsurgical dietary program. It is important for patients to follow the dietary program prescribed by their surgeon and/or program. If a patient is not given a postsurgical dietary program, he or she may wish to discuss with his or her surgeon, program nurse, or dietitian the possibility of working through these five-phases.

Phase One: A clear liquid diet that begins after surgery. The purpose of phase one is to allow for the secure healing of the stomach and reattachments of the intestine. It provides an oral source of fluid and a small number of calories and electrolytes as a means of preventing dehydration.

Phase Two: A full liquid dietary program that begins when the patient demonstrates the ability to tolerate fluids. This phase adds a protein supplement to the clear liquids included in phase one. The supplement is added to meet more of the nutritional needs of the body.

Phase Three: This phase adds foods of a creamy consistency to the diet. It provides a greater variety of foods and a more complete form of nutrition.

Phase Four: Foods of a pureed or blenderized consistency are added to the diet. Pureed or blenderized foods are easy to digest. They also pass easily through the restrictive band or ring used in some weight loss surgery procedures.

Phase Five: Patients should be able to eat solid foods by phase five. Portion sizes for meals are typically quite small and patients are advised to continue taking a protein supplement, juices, and clear fluids between meals.

The time frame for working through the five phases will vary from patient to patient and surgery to surgery. Some surgeons have patients move through these phases in a few days or weeks. Others space them out over a two to three month period.

The stomach pouch will gradually stretch to hold more food than it could hold just after surgery (except, perhaps, for the Adjustable Lap Band or Silastic Ring VSG, *aka* Fobi Pouch). Patients are advised to increase consumption as they can tolerate more food. It is not unusual for it to take up to six months after surgery to reach the maximum pouch consumption capacity. Consumption capacity will vary somewhat with combined restrictive/malabsorptive procedures having a capacity of about one cup

Five-Phase Dietary Program

63

per meal. Mostly malabsorptive procedures may allow patients to consume small to average size meals.

LIVING COMFORTABLY WITH A WEIGHT LOSS SURGERY PROCEDURE

Living Comfortably with your Surgical Tool

In addition to following the food phases, several other factors have been found helpful for protecting and living comfortably with a weight loss surgery procedure. Constipation is a common experience restrictive and combined restrictive/malabsorptive procedure patients have due to decreased consumption and decreased bulk or fiber in the diet. While the schedule of bowel movements may be permanently changed, it is important to avoid constipation. If constipation does occur during the first four dietary phases, patients may be advised to use Mineral Oil, Milk of Magnesia, Laci LeBeau's Super Dieters Tea or one cup of warm water into which the juice of half a lemon has been squeezed. From phase five on, any of the above may be used, or one-half of a graham cracker may be eaten. High fiber products for constipation are not to be used.

Food tolerance may be significantly affected by the reduced size of the stomach and how well the eating guidelines presented above are followed. Though food tolerance or intolerance is highly individual there are some foods that most patients do not eat comfortably following restrictive or combined procedures. These include fibrous meats such as steak, doughy breads, some raw fruits and vegetables, fruit and vegetable skin, and foods that are very fatty. Once intolerable foods are identified, it is best to avoid them. Eating foods that are not tolerated may lead to vomiting. In procedures that create a stapled pouch that is not divided from the larger stomach, chronic vomiting may eventually weaken the staple line and result in staple line leak or failure. When this happens patients are hungry more often and can eat larger portions of food, contributing to weight regain. Food tolerance is supported by following the eating behavior guidelines carefully. Food is to be eaten in small bites and pureed in the mouth before swallowing.

Some patients have noted that the order in which they eat foods makes a difference in food tolerance. These patients recommend that food be eaten in order of softness with the foods that liquefy or digest most quickly being

64

eaten first. Foods that are solid and digest more slowly are best eaten last. As an example, a patient might eat these foods in this order: Jell-O®, mashed potato, vegetables, meat, and bread.

For maximum weight loss, patients are advised to limit daily calorie consumption. For patients who have had a restrictive or restrictive/malabsorptive procedure, calorie consumption varies between 800 and 1400+ calories depending on the program and patient needs. Daily calorie consumption for patients who have had a malabsorptive procedure may be much higher. It is very important that a nutritionally balanced diet be consumed. Patients are also advised to take a chewable or liquid vitamin daily. Working with the multidisciplinary team, each patient's specific calorie intake can be monitored and adjustments made to insure good nutrition. The multidisciplinary team will also help the patient design a maintenance calorie and nutritional program when the goal weight has been reached.

SPECIAL CONSIDERATIONS FOR PATIENTS WITH RESTRICTIVE PROCEDURES

Following a restrictive procedure or those using a silastic ring, food must always be chewed carefully and eaten slowly. When food is not eaten carefully enough, it may get caught in or "plug up" the ring. It is clear that this has happened when the pouch is full and does not empty. The patient may feel discomfort and will not be able to eat or drink anything additional. Vomiting may also occur.

If something does get stuck, surgeons have several remedies they may recommend (*e.g.*, Mineral Oil) to cause the food to slip through the ring. If these methods do not work, it may be necessary for a procedure called an endoscopy to be ordered to clear the ring. During an endoscopy, a patient is mildly sedated and a tube is inserted down the esophagus into the pouch to clear the ring.

Patients who take medication are advised to take it in a liquid form, if it is available. If no liquid form is available, pills should be crushed, cut, or chewed, in order to avoid becoming stuck in the ring. Once the stomach is completely healed, medication may usually be swallowed whole if it is no larger than the

Special Considerations for Patients with Restrictive Procedures

size of an Advil. If there are any questions with regard to how a medication should be taken, the prescribing physician should be consulted.

SPECIAL CONSIDERATIONS FOR COMBINED RESTRICTIVE AND/OR MALABSORPTIVE PROCEDURES

A pill becoming stuck is not a concern for patients who have had a combined procedure that does not include a silastic ring. However, for the first month after surgery, they are advised to crush or chew any pills taken. Approximately one month after surgery, gastric bypass patients may begin to swallow pills whole. Patients are encouraged to swallow pills one at a time. Special questions about taking medication should be directed to the prescribing physician.

Combined procedure patients must always be concerned about limiting their intake of sugar in order to avoid the dumping syndrome. Patients who have had a mainly malabsorptive procedure must limit fat consumption in order to avoid diarrhea. They must also be especially diligent in taking their vitamins and making sure they get sufficient amounts of vitamin B12, calcium and iron. Here again, the prescribing physician can best advise the patient about the precise amount of these supplements to be taken.

Mindy

I am a gastroplasty patient. My surgery was done May 10, 1993, and I have never regretted making that decision. My lifestyle growing up with three brothers and sisters in a single parent home only allowed for a high fat, high volume diet. Unfortunately, my diet didn't change when I became an adult. I chose to be an insecure person that ignored my weight problem by spending most of my time in my own safe, comfortable world. I was truly blind to what my diet was doing to me and my body.

When I reached 323 pounds I could no longer ignore my problem. I could no longer walk without cortisone injections to the heels of my feet. My knees were getting worse by the day. For five years I wanted a second child very badly. But I was told I would never be able to carry a pregnancy to term without a lot of complications. I had gotten to the point that because of my size, my embarrassment, and my pain, I could no longer go about my normal daily routine like nothing was wrong with me. Even in the best of situations, there was someone around who would remind me I was not normal, something was wrong with me. I felt like a robot who was mechanical on the inside yet had skin, eyes, etc. on the outside. Finally I malfunctioned, thanks be to God.

I went to see my husband's family internist. He carefully explained to me the procedure of vertical stapled gastroplasty and referred me to a surgical program. After consultation, I decided to have gastroplasty. The program's patient coordinator helped me get the ball rolling with my insurance provider and completing the necessary paper work. She helped me find my surgeon.

To date I have lost eighty pounds and so many inches I have lost count. I am down six dress sizes. With the help of my support group, I can now nurture myself mentally to help my weight loss. I have started to become all the things I've always dreamed of being... Confident, Secure, and Strong. I have a direction in my life now. I can see the light at the end of the tunnel. I am in control.

Gastroplasty has been a second chance and more. It is like being reborn with all the new and innocent organs and features of an infant. I am waiting to see what becomes of this new life of mine. I know I will be able to rewrite my past lifestyle as far as food goes. I feel that my remaining years on this earth are now going to be Happy, Healthy, and Good Looking ones. I have self-esteem and a feeling of belonging that I never had before.

Everyone connected to my program has been committed and sincere. They have been consistent in helping me make my second chance an incredible and exciting adventure. My love and thanks to everyone in the program, the doctors, staff and all my new friends at group. ❧

CHAPTER FIVE

Eating for Health, Weight Loss and Maintenance

Funk and Wagnalls *New International Dictionary of the English Language* defines the word 'food' as "That which is eaten or drunk or absorbed for the growth and repair of organisms and the maintenance of life... That which increases, keeps active, or sustains."

Food is a good thing. It keeps us alive.

Food is a good thing for many other reasons, as well. Food provides pleasure to all of our senses. We enjoy the way it looks, tastes, smells, and feels. Food provides opportunities for social interaction. We share food when we do business, to strengthen the bonds of family and friendship, to encourage romance. The kinds of foods we buy and where we buy or eat them can give us a sense of power, affluence, or social status. Cooking food can provide an exciting career or be a creative outlet. We use food as a reward or for the purpose of celebration. And food comforts us in times of illness or distress.

Food is a good thing. But there is an old cliché about too much of a good thing. Too much of a good thing can be a bad thing. In the case of food, too much of it can lead to severe obesity and poor physical health. This, in turn, can lead to depression, self-hatred and the fear of others. It can limit or deprive us of personal, interpersonal, educational, recreational, and career goals.

Those who are overweight know well the bad things brought on by eating too much food. Day in and day out, they wage a war with food. They usually do this by dieting. But diets seldom work. Though they might win a battle, they ultimately lose the war.

For the severely obese, weight loss surgeries are tools for making peace with food. The restriction on consumption or malabsorption makes it difficult, though not impossible, to eat enough food to maintain obesity. The procedures maximize the good things food can bring to life and minimize the bad.

Following weight loss surgery, it is important that a patient develop a positive relationship with food. They must learn about good nutrition and eating to sustain health. They must learn to make food choices that will protect the stomach pouch and encourage weight loss and maintenance. This chapter will discuss the basics of good nutrition. It will tell how to choose and enjoy a healthy weight loss and maintenance diet.

THE BASICS OF GOOD NUTRITION…

Today many people are confused about nutrition, and with good reason. Almost daily we read or hear about a new scientific study that suggests we should or should not eat a certain food. Following weight loss surgery, patients don't have to become an expert in nutrition. However, it is important to learn a few basics about healthful eating. First it is important to know just what food is.

Food is a material that consists essentially of three ingredients: Protein, carbohydrate and fat. A calorie is a unit of measurement that indicates how much energy or fuel each of these ingredients provides to the body. Choosing a healthy diet means knowing about these three ingredients and how much of them the body needs.

Aside from water, protein is the most abundant material in the body. It is a basic building block that benefits the body by carrying oxygen in the blood, building muscle and all other body tissue, and building the enzymes that digest food. Protein is used to build DNA, which provides the genes with the code necessary to transmit heredity. It is part of insulin and helps to regulate blood sugar levels.

The Recommended Daily Allowance (RDA) of protein is 44 grams for an adult woman and 56 grams for an adult man. Each gram of protein provides the body with 4½ calories of energy. Foods rich in protein are lean meats, fish, eggs, low fat dairy products, legumes such as peas and lentils, and all kinds of beans.

Carbohydrate is the basic fuel for the body. It comes in three forms: *simple*, *double*, and *complex*. All three types of carbohydrate break down into sugar. Simple sugar is fuel that may be directly used for energy. The body processes must break down double and complex carbohydrates into simple sugar before they are used for fuel.

The RDA of carbohydrate for an adult is 125 grams. All types of carbohydrate provide the body with 4½ calories of energy per gram. Double and complex carbohydrates are found in foods such as cereal, pasta, rice and bread and in many vegetables. Simple carbohydrates are found in sugar, honey, jam and jelly, candy and other sweetened foods.

Fat is a highly concentrated source of fuel for the body that is especially beneficial for endurance activities. Fat is necessary to help the body absorb many nutrients. Among these are carotene and vitamins A, D, E, and K. Fat provides the body with essential fatty acids. It protects the vital organs and prevents heat loss. As a concentrated form of energy, fat contains nine calories of energy per gram.

The RDA of fat for an adult is presented in a range. It is recommended that adults limit their intake of fat to between 15 to 30 percent of their daily calorie intake. Fat is contained in various amounts in protein and carbohydrate foods. In high concentration, fat is found in butter, oils and lard, and products made primarily of these ingredients, like salad dressing.

In addition to the protein, carbohydrate, and fat described above, food also provides two other important nutritional ingredients: Vitamins and minerals. Vitamins are organic substances (nutrients derived from living sources such as plants and animals) that the body requires in small amounts to support the processes of life. Vitamins are agents of change, also known as catalysts, which cause chemical reactions among other nutrients to assure that the functions of the body are operating smoothly. The role of vitamins is preventative. When consumed in the recommended amounts, vitamins prevent the body from being susceptible to any of the vitamin deficiency diseases (such as scurvy, which is caused by a lack of Vitamin C). With the exception of Vitamin D (the sunshine vitamin), the body does not produce its own vitamins. Vitamins must be obtained from the food that is consumed.

Minerals are inorganic nutrients such as materials that are mined from the earth. Minerals are required by the body in small amounts and are found in many food sources. Minerals fulfill their function by actually becoming part of the body structure. The skeleton and teeth are made largely of calcium. Iron is a chief component in red blood cells.

The FDA has established an RDA for both vitamins and minerals. Most healthy people obtain the vitamins and minerals they need by consuming a variety of foods and beverages. Those who consume less than 1800 calories a day and/or whose diet is inadequate in its variety, often benefit by taking a multivitamin daily.

THE SOURCE OF GOOD NUTRITION...

Prior to 1992 the source of good nutrition was considered to be the Four Basic Food Groups. These four food groups were dairy products; vegetables and fruits; meat, fish and poultry; and beans and grains. Each food group was considered to be equal to the others. It was recommended that people eat an equal number of servings of food from each group on a daily basis.

Now we have learned that the foods in these four groups are not equal. We know that some foods provide more or better nutrition to the body than others. In 1992, the United States Department of Agriculture (USDA) replaced the Four Basic Food Groups with the Food Pyramid.

In the Food Pyramid, the emphasis is on eating from the bottom up. Most of our calories are to be consumed in the form of complex carbohydrates (foods made from grains), followed by vegetables and fruits; dairy products; meats, fish, and poultry; with the least of our calories consumed in fat and simple carbohydrates (sugar).

The USDA recommends a range of servings per day for each food group on the Pyramid. The servings recommended cover a wide range of body sizes and activity levels. The smaller and less active a person is, the lower the number of servings they should eat. The larger and more active a person is, the higher number of servings they should eat.

GOOD NUTRITION DURING WEIGHT LOSS

Before having weight loss surgery most patients consumed a high volume, high calorie diet. Though patients may have eaten too much food, leading to obesity and its related health issues, they were probably eating more than enough protein, carbohydrate, and fat to nourish their body. Also contained in the food consumed were all the vitamins and minerals necessary to meet daily requirements.

Weight loss surgeries dramatically restrict the volume of food that can be consumed or results in some malabsorption of calories and nutrients contained in the food that is eaten. Because consumption is restricted and/or calories and nutrients are malabsorbed, it is vitally important that patients eat a nutritious diet following their procedure in order to provide the body with the energy and building blocks it needs to be healthy.

Sally Myers, a Registered Dietitian with considerable experience in treating weight loss surgery patients, has revised the USDA Food Pyramid to illustrate the diet her research suggests is appropriate for weight loss surgery patients. (*See figure 10*) In her *Food Pyramid for the Weight Loss Surgery Patient*, protein foods replace grains as the foundation of the diet. Restrictive and combined/restrictive patients should consume the smaller number of servings and the more malabsorptive patients should consume the larger number of servings noted on the pyramid.

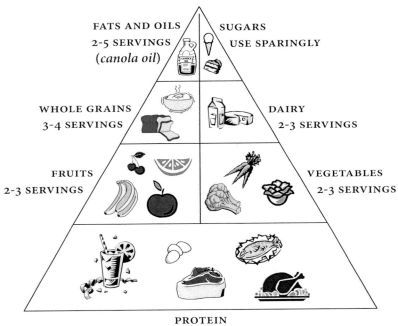

FATS AND OILS
2-5 SERVINGS
(canola oil)

SUGARS
USE SPARINGLY

WHOLE GRAINS
3-4 SERVINGS

DAIRY
2-3 SERVINGS

FRUITS
2-3 SERVINGS

VEGETABLES
2-3 SERVINGS

PROTEIN
3-5 SERVINGS
(meats, legumes, soy, protein drinks)

Figure 10 – *Food Pyramid modified for the Gastric Bypass Patient*
(after Sally Myers)

What is a serving? Sally Myers gives the following guidelines for serving sizes:

Protein:
2 to 3 ounces of beef, poultry, fish, or pork (skin removed)
½ cup of legumes (black, kidney, navy, pinto beans)
1 ounce of low-fat or non-fat cheese
1 egg
¼ cup nuts or seeds
2 tablespoons of peanut butter
1 cup of 1% or skim (non-fat) milk

Sally recommends patients consume between 70 and 120 grams of protein daily. Malabsorptive procedure patients may need to consume more. Also at least 40 grams of the protein consumed should be in animal, whey, or soy products.

Complex
Carbohydrates:
(Starches)
1 slice of whole grain bread
1 corn tortilla
1 slice of thin crust pizza (widest part is 2 inches)
½ whole grain bagel or English muffin
¼ cup brown rice, pasta, or hot cereal

Fruit:
½ or whole (small sized) apple, peach, plum, nectarine
¼ to ½ cup of sliced or diced fruit
4 ounces of fruit juice

Vegetables:
¼ to ½ cup cooked vegetables
½ to 1 cup raw vegetables
6 ounces of vegetable juice (low sodium)

Dairy:
1 cup of 1% or non-fat milk or soy milk
½ to 1 cup cottage cheese
1 ounce of low fat cheese
½ to 1 cup of low-fat or non-fat yogurt

Fats: 2 to 5 teaspoons daily

Fats consumed should provide the body with the essential fatty acids needed for the absorption of the fat-soluble vitamins and to protect against fatty acid deficiency. Good sources of fatty acids are safflower oil, sunflower oil, corn oil, soybean oil, cottonseed oil, canola oil, salmon, tuna, and sardines.

Sugars: Use sparingly

Immediately after weight loss surgery and continuing until the patient achieves maximum possible weight loss, the number of calories consumed should support weight loss. Dr. C. Everett Koop, former Surgeon General of the United States and founder of Shape Up America, in association with the American Obesity Association, recommends a core treatment option for weight reduction for all weight loss programs. This core treatment option involves a moderate deficit diet of 1200+ calories a day for women and 1400+ calories a day for men. A number of weight loss programs, including those utilizing weight loss surgery, use the moderate deficit diet. Others use a low-calorie diet of 800 to 1200 calories per day for women and 800 to 1400 calories per day for men to encourage more rapid weight loss. Patients who have had a mainly malabsorptive procedure often require significantly more calories than listed above.

It is important that the nutritional needs of each weight loss surgery patient be evaluated on a somewhat individual basis. In general, patients are advised to consume at least 100 grams of carbohydrate (approximately 450 calories) and between 10 and 30 grams of fat (approximately 90 to 270 calories) daily. Protein is often calculated for each patient based on Ideal Body Weight (IBW):

IBW *Daily Protein Intake Formula*

Step One: Determine IBW by…
                   Female: Start with a base weight of 100 pounds for the first 5 feet in height, add 5 pounds for every additional inch in height above 5 feet.
                   Example: 5´5″ female = 125 LBS IBW (10% more or less may be calculated for body frame)
                   Male: Start with a base weight of 106 pounds for the first 5 feet in height, add 6 pounds for every additional inch in height above 5 feet.
                   Example: 5´10″ male = 172 LBS IBW (10% more or less may be calculated for body frame)

Step Two: Convert IBW to kilograms (kg) by dividing IBW by 2.2…
                   125 LBS IBW 2.2 = 56 kg IBW
                   172 LBS IBW divided by 2.2 = 78 kg IBW

Step One: Determine IBW by…
                   56 kg × 0.8 = approximately 45 grams of protein per day (about 200 calories)
                   78 kg × 0.8 = approximately 62 grams of protein per day (about 280 calories)

Patti Pedrick, another Registered Dietitian experienced in treating weight loss surgery patients, suggests that women over 300 pounds, men over 350 pounds, and patients who have had a mainly malabsorptive procedure, often require more protein than that provided by the IBW calculation. She recommends using the Adjusted Body Weight (ABW) formula to calculate daily protein intake for these patients.

Good Nutrition during Weight Loss

ABW *Daily Protein Intake Formula*

Step One: Use Step One of the IBW formula to determine a reference ideal body weight.

Step Two: Subtract reference body weight from actual body weight.

Step Three: Divide the answer by 4 and add the answer to the reference body weight.

Step Four: Divide this number by 2.2 to determine weight in kilograms (kg).

Step Five: Multiply the answer by 1.5 to determine the number of grams of protein to be consumed daily.

Examples:

Female:
5′ 4″ with a weight of 325 LBS
325—120 = 205 LBS
205 ÷ 4 = 51
51 + 120 = 171
171 ÷ 2.2 = 78 kg
78 × 1.5 = 117 grams of protein (about 526 calories)

Male:
5′ 11″ with a weight of 425 LBS
425—189 = 236 LBS
236 ÷ 4 = 59
59 + 189 = 248
248 ÷ 2.2 = 113 kg
113 × 1.5 = 169.5 grams of protein (about 763 calories)

In order to avoid consuming more protein than necessary, daily protein intake should be recalculated using either formula after every 30 pounds of weight loss.

A sample daily menu during weight loss may include:

Breakfast

3 OZ	nonfat milk
1 OZ	ready to eat cereal
2 OZ	orange juice

Morning Snack

1 OZ	string cheese
3	graham crackers
3 OZ	nonfat milk

Lunch

Fresh vegetables such as cucumber slices, radishes and carrots
1 Tuna fish sandwich with:

	1 TSP mayonnaise
	¼ cup (2 OZ) tuna, and
	2 slices of bread
3 OZ	nonfat milk

Afternoon Snack

4-6	saltine crackers
15	grapes
3 OZ	nonfat milk

Dinner

2 OZ	chicken
2 OZ	potato
2 OZ	green beans
1 TSP	margarine

Evening Snack

¼ cup	(2 oz) cottage cheese
3 oz	nonfat milk
1 oz	fresh vegetables such as jicama, carrots, cucumber
Plus:	8 oz fruit juice and approximately 64 oz non-caloric beverages per day (water, diet drinks, tea, etc.) Low-calorie juice and water may be added between meals in order to provide the body with all the fluids needed for health.

For patients who are not provided with a dietary plan or who wish to design their own, the following guidelines may be useful in helping them consume a well balanced diet:

Protein:	25 to 35 percent of total daily caloric intake.
Carbohydrate:	40 to 60 percent of total daily caloric intake (at least 100 grams).
Fat:	10 to 20 percent of total daily caloric intake.

Several special issues are important to consider regarding the nutritional program for weight loss following bariatric surgery. First, patients who have had one of the malabsorptive procedures typically require more protein and calories than those who have had restrictive or restrictive/malabsorptive procedures. This is because the malabsorptive procedures bypass a longer portion of the small intestine, increasing malabsorption. Second, some weight loss surgery programs recommend that patients eat three meals per day and avoid snacking. The concern is that snacking, or eating several mini-meals per day, may encourage overeating. If the stomach pouch is large enough to consume the amount of food included in the nutritional plan in three meals, this is an appropriate option. Third, some patients find that they do not have the pouch volume needed to consume all the food on the nutritional plan even in several mini-meals. If this is true, members of the multidisciplinary treatment team should be prepared to make suggestions about how to increase protein and/or calorie consumption without increasing volume.

When a patient has reached goal weight, it is necessary to adjust their daily calorie intake from a weight loss level to a weight maintenance level. It usually takes between 11 and 18 calories to support each pound of body weight. The actual number of calories needed to support one pound of body weight depends upon a person's basal metabolic rate (BMR) and activity level. Both affect the rate at which calories are burned as fuel.

For most restrictive or combined/restrictive patients, a maintenance calorie intake may be calculated using a daily consumption of 11 calories per pound of body weight. As an example, suppose a patient has reached a goal weight of 130 pounds. To find their maintenance daily calorie intake, 130 pounds is multiplied by 11 calories to reach the number 1450. This means, the patient could conceivably eat 1450 calories per day and maintain the goal weight of 130 pounds.

If the patient's BMR is low or if their lifestyle is sedentary, 1450 calories per day may be too many and they may begin to regain weight. Should this happen, the patient would need to decrease calorie intake until a maintenance level is identified. As an example, should the patient gain weight by eating 11 calories per pound per day, they would need to decrease calorie intake until their weight stabilized at 130 pounds. Let us say they discovered that they could eat 9 calories per pound per day to maintain a goal of 130 pounds. Multiplying 130 by 9 gives a daily intake of 1170 calories.

Conversely, let us say the patient had a normal BMR and exercised for one hour every day. At 1450 calories per day, they continue to lose weight and drop below the goal weight of 130 pounds. Since continued weight loss may damage health, it is important to stop further weight loss. The patient would need to gradually increase daily calorie intake until they stabilized their weight at 130 pounds. If they found that they stabilized their weight by eating 14 calories per pound each day, using the formula above, they would need to eat 1820 calories per day to maintain the goal weight.

Restrictive and combined/restricted surgeries permanently restrict the volume of food that can be consumed at one time. It will not be possible to adjust from a weight loss to a weight maintenance diet by increasing the amount of food eaten. Instead of eating more food, it will be necessary to increase the calorie content of the foods eaten. This is usually done by increasing the fat

Good Nutrition for Weight Maintenance...

81

content of the foods eaten. Once on a maintenance diet, a patient may drink low-fat milk rather than non-fat milk. Since fat has twice as many calories as protein and carbohydrate, calorie content can be increased dramatically by slightly increasing the fat content of the foods eaten. A sample menu for one day might include the following:

Breakfast

2 TBLSP	Cream of Wheat
2 TBLSP	low-fat milk
1 TBLSP	applesauce
1 TSP	margarine

Mid-morning Snack

1 OZ	low-fat cottage cheese
¼ slice	bread
2 TBLSP	apricots

Lunch

1 OZ	chicken
2 TBLSP	mashed potato
2 TBLSP	cooked carrots
2 TBLSP	banana
1 TSP	margarine

Mid-afternoon snack

1 OZ	low-fat yogurt
¼ slice	bread
1 OZ	banana

Dinner

1 OZ	fish
2 TBLSP	angel hair pasta
2 TBLSP	peas
2 TBLSP	strawberries
1 TSP	margarine

Unlike the restrictive and combined restrictive/malabsorptive procedures, the malabsorptive procedures do not dramatically restrict the amount of food a patient can consume. After healing, BPD and BPD/DS patients may not consume the large amounts of foods eaten before surgery, but they can eat almost normal size portions of food. Malabsorptive procedure patients may find that a higher daily calorie intake is needed to stop weight loss once they have reached their goal weight.

Once a weight loss surgery patient has determined the number of calories required to stabilize their weight, the calories consumed should be portioned according to the guidelines for protein, carbohydrates, fats and sugars provided above.

A SPECIAL WORD ABOUT VITAMINS...

As stated above, the reduced size of the stomach following weight loss surgery makes it difficult for patients to consume the calories necessary to provide the body with the RDA of vitamins and minerals. Taking a multivitamin supplement daily becomes vitally important to protecting the health of weight loss surgery patients. Expensive vitamin supplements are not necessary. Most commonly sold, over-the-counter, brands are acceptable.

A multivitamin a day is usually sufficient for restrictive procedure patients. Combined restrictive/malabsorptive and malabsorptive procedure patients generally require additional vitamin supplementation. They often need additional vitamin B12, folic acid and calcium. Women who have menstrual cycles also require additional iron. The amounts of these additional supplements are typically as follows:

Vitamin B12:   500 mcg daily or 1 mg injection monthly
Folic Acid: 400 mcg daily
Calcium: 1000 mg daily
Iron: 25 mg or 325 mg of ferrous sulfate (another form of iron)

Vitamin B12 is necessary for the building of genetic material, the formation of red blood cells, and the functioning of the nervous system. Folic acid is a member of the B vitamin family and helps form body proteins and genetic material and is involved in the formation of hemoglobin. Calcium and iron are minerals. Calcium is important for hard bones and blood clotting, and to activate a number of enzymes. Iron transports and transfers oxygen in blood and tissues and is part of hemoglobin in blood, myoglobin in muscles, protoplasm of cells, cell nuclei, and many enzymes and tissues.

Malabsorptive procedure patients may require even more of the supplements described above because of the longer bypass of the small intestine and increased malabsorption. Supplementation of the fat-soluble vitamins A, D, E, and K is common. Other vitamins and minerals, such as zinc, may be prescribed as needed.

To determine the need for an adjustment in the amount of protein, vitamins, and minerals a patient may require, surgeons who do weight loss surgery may request blood tests. For the average patient, blood tests may be done at six months following surgery, again at one year following surgery, and then yearly. Patients with special health and/or medical issues may benefit from more frequent monitoring.

THE IMPORTANCE OF WATER...

Earlier it was mentioned that protein is the second most abundant material in the body. The most abundant material is water. And water is vitally important to health. We will die much sooner from the lack of water than we will from the lack of food.

Drinking sufficient water becomes especially important following weight loss surgery for several reasons. First, most foods that we eat are comprised of a high percentage of water. Most fruits and vegetables are between 80 and 90 percent water. Chicken and beef contain, on average, about 60 percent water. Cheddar cheese is approximately 37 percent, and chocolate cake is approximately 25 percent water. The water in these foods may help to hydrate the body.

Because of the reduced food consumption following weight loss surgery, a patient will not get as much of the water needed by the body from food. The result is increased thirst. Drinking water in its purest form is the best way

84

to hydrate the body and eliminate thirst. It may be interesting to note that many cravings for food are really a sign of thirst, not hunger. By drinking sufficient water, the weight loss surgery patient will keep the body hydrated, and decrease the craving for food.

Another reason water is so important is that it assists the body in getting rid of excess fat. In order for fat to be lost from the body, it must first be oxidized. Through the oxidation process, carbon dioxide and water are formed. The carbon dioxide is rapidly eliminated from the body during exhalation. The water must travel through the body until it reaches the bladder to be excreted. By drinking plenty of water, a patient provides the body with the fluid necessary to get rid of the oxidized fat through urination.

The Importance of Water...

How much water is recommended? We all know the formula of eight, eight ounce glasses per day (64 ounces). Right after surgery, when the stomach is at its smallest, drinking this much water might be impossible. It is recommended, however, that patients suck on ice chips or sip water frequently. As the stomach heals and stretches to its greatest capacity, drinking 64 ounces of water per day will become easier. Since patients are never able to drink liquids quickly following the procedure, it is recommended that they carry a water bottle with them and sip from it throughout the day.

The emphasis here is on water… straight. Drinking other beverages does not provide the hydration the body needs. Caffeinated and alcoholic beverages act as diuretics and may dehydrate the body. Fluids like regular soda or fruit and vegetable juice have many calories and may lead to weight gain. Any of these beverages should be consumed in moderation. Alcoholic beverages should be consumed with considerable care and caution. Many patients report that they become intoxicated much more quickly following weight loss surgery than they did before. Don't like the taste of straight water? Take a tip from fine restaurants and add a slice of lemon for flavor.

DEVELOPING A NEW RELATIONSHIP WITH FOOD…

Weight loss surgery patients report interesting reactions to food following the procedure. Some can't tolerate an association with food beyond that of taking in the nutrition they need as dictated by their food phase. They don't like going to the market. They don't like preparing food. They don't like to watch other people eat. The very thought of these activities brings feelings of sadness, frustration, anger, or repulsion. To them, food continues to be a bad thing. These reactions are usually temporary and suggestions for dealing with them will be discussed in a later chapter.

Some patients report that they enjoy their interaction with food more than ever before. Trips to the market are an adventure. They watch cooking shows on television and pore over recipes. They cook large amounts of food and, though they can't eat it, enjoy watching others eat what they have prepared. There is greater enjoyment of the foods they do eat.

Food really is a good thing. It is important to remember that following weight loss surgery, eating doesn't have to be boring or tasteless. All the good things about food mentioned earlier in this chapter can be a part of the eating experience. With careful nutritional planning, favorite foods, restaurants, and social functions can be enjoyed. Cooking and eating food can still be a creative outlet. And food can provide comfort and nurture in many healthful ways. It just won't take so much food to provide pleasure and satisfaction. Be willing to develop a more positive attitude about your relationship with food.

A WORD ABOUT FOOD CRAVINGS...

The ability to distinguish between hunger and fullness is described by the term *Interoceptive Awareness*. Before weight loss surgery, many patients rarely, if ever, felt real physical hunger. Many rarely, if ever, felt a sense of satiety (sense of fullness and satisfaction). Bariatric surgery often enables a patient to experience interoceptive awareness. It can be exciting to experience the control of eating only when physically hungry and stopping when comfortably satisfied.

To eat in a way that meets the nutritional needs of the body and supports weight loss and/or maintenance, it is important to eat only when physically hungry and stop eating when comfortably full. It is also important to be able to distinguish between physical hunger, biological hunger, and emotional hunger. Biological hunger and emotional hunger are best known as cravings.

In the book *Why Women Need Chocolate*, Debra Waterhouse, MPH, RD, gives the following tips for determining between these three feelings of hunger:

Physical Hunger: Both the stomach and the brain send clear signals that they are lacking the energy food supplies to help the body and brain function efficiently. When a person is physically hungry the stomach growls, pangs, and has a hollow or empty feeling. The brain signals hunger by being foggy, unable to concentrate, getting a headache, or feeling fatigue. The average person gets physically hungry every 4 to 5 hours. Eating a well-balanced, appropriately sized meal will satisfy the hunger and provide the energy the body and brain needs to function.

A Word about Food Cravings...

Biological Hunger: Biological hunger or cravings occur when the body or brain needs something. Physical hunger always precedes biological cravings. A person is experiencing biological hunger if he or she is physically hungry, the hunger intensifies over time and the hunger is accompanied by a negative mood (such as being sad, angry, anxious, stressed, tired). When biological hunger is experienced, eating a *small amount* of the food craved will generally satisfy the hunger, end the craving, and improve the mood.

Emotional Hunger: In contrast to physical or biological hunger, emotional hunger is not preceded by physical hunger. A person is experiencing emotional hunger if the craving does not intensify over time but the negative mood does intensify over time. Eating the craved food (even in large amounts) does not satisfy the craving or improve the mood. Typically, emotional hunger is only satisfied when the emotional need is met. It is important to identify the emotional need and take action to satisfy it.

HEALTH ALERT...

The bottom line for all patients following weight loss surgery is to learn to protect their health and weight loss by following a nutritious eating program. Poor nutrition can eventually lead to poor health. Poor food choices can lead to weight regain.

To protect from weight regain, a nutritious diet with a limited fat intake should be eaten. Foods high in fat and sugar (and calories) liquefy very quickly. As foods liquefy they leave the stomach pouch and enter the intestines to continue the digestive process. An empty stomach pouch can lead to hunger and/or make it possible to engage in frequent snacking. These activities stop weight loss or promote weight regain.

A healthy diet of low-fat, low-sugar carbohydrates and proteins takes a long time to digest. These foods stay in the stomach pouch and keep it full for a longer time than fat or simple sugar foods. Eating low-fat, low-sugar carbohydrates and proteins nourishes the body and decreases cravings and hunger. A stomach pouch that is full of healthy foods eliminates the need for, or possibility of, frequent snacking.

Hair loss, low energy, muscle cramping or pain, depression and irritability are a few side affects of poor nutrition. Patients who experience these, or any other distressing physical or mental symptoms, should consult a physician immediately. Failure to do so may seriously place one's health at risk. Simple nutritional adjustments and the addition of food supplements may be all that is necessary to end these symptoms and improve health.

Tammy

To describe what vertical stapled gastroplasty has meant to me is very hard to do in just a few sentences. When my counselor and patient coordinator say gastroplasty is only a tool, that is the truth. We all would love to have a miracle cure for our obesity, but the truth is it takes work and determination. Gastroplasty is not a miracle cure. But I can say that along with Jesus and my husband, Gary, gastroplasty saved my life!

I was on a suicidal course. I weighed two hundred forty pounds totally naked! This was a vast difference from the one hundred ten pounds I weighed when I got married. To go into all the reasons why I allowed myself to balloon up to two hundred forty pounds would take a whole book. I can tell you that I spent thousands of dollars trying every diet, and even counseling, trying to lose weight. I came to the point in my life at 32 years old, a wife and mother of three precious children, that I knew I was only going to continue to gain weight if I didn't get some kind of help. My problem was that horrible hungry feeling you get on a diet. That feeling would make me want to climb a wall.

To make gastroplasty sound easy would be a lie. This is a major surgery. In my opinion it is definitely not for everyone. I knew that this was going to be my last chance to have a healthy and fulfilled life. This decision would be a life long decision. The first two months after surgery were horrible. I was a real ugly person to live with. I could have never gone through it without the support of a loving husband.

Now that seven months have gone by I would do it all over again in a heartbeat. I'm not at my goal of one hundred thirty pounds yet. But for the first time in a long time, I know my dream is going to come true. In the meantime, gastroplasty has taken away that horrible hungry feeling I got while dieting. It has given me a chance to run and play with my children. It has given me a chance to live again. ❧

CHAPTER SIX

Exercising for Weight Loss and Maintenance

It is hard to escape the bombardment of information on the importance of exercise to overall health. It is promoted on television, in magazines, and in newspapers. There are literally hundreds of exercise books and videos available. There are numerous gyms and fitness centers in every community. In spite of its reported importance and the number of programs available, the truth is very few people follow the advice of the Nike commercial and "just do it."

According to a study by the US Public Health Service, only about 20 percent of all Americans exercise consistently enough to get any benefit from doing it. Among the remaining 80 percent, half exercise occasionally and half don't exercise at all. Those who don't exercise regularly always have an excuse… "I'm too busy or tired…" "I don't have the money to join a fitness center…" "My family needs me at home when they are home…" "I don't have the proper clothing or equipment…" "Exercising is boring…" "I hate to get all sweaty and smelly."

Perhaps the most common reason why people don't exercise is that they do it inappropriately. A woman may join an aerobics class. Although it is her first time to attend, she works out as hard as she can and finishes the whole one-hour exercise session. A man may join a gym and insist that he begin his program at a level that takes his muscles past the point of "the burn." After all, everyone has heard the slogan, "No pain... no gain!" And the immediate result for both is just that... pain. Pain that is so intense the possibility of continuing any form of exercise is unthinkable.

Relax, for there is good news! Exercise does not have to be painful, grim, or punishing to be beneficial. For good cardiovascular conditioning and weight maintenance, exercise just needs to be done consistently. For weight loss, exercise needs to be done consistently and for a specified amount of time.

This chapter will clarify the relationship of exercise to weight loss and maintenance. The benefits of regular exercise will be presented. Exercise tips for the weight loss surgery will also be given.

THE RELATIONSHIP BETWEEN EXERCISE, EATING, AND WEIGHT...

Mark Bricklin is the author of *Lose Weight Naturally*. In his book, he asks this question, "Most people who are overweight eat too darn much. True or False?"

The answer is False! The truth is that some people who are overweight do eat too much. But most people who are overweight do not. In fact, many overweight people actually eat less than average weight people do.

How is this possible? Bricklin explains this seeming paradox. He reports that several large population studies were done comparing the eating habits of normal weight to overweight (not obese) people. The results of the studies indicate that, while average weight and overweight people may eat the same number of calories, average weight people are more physically active. They burn in activity all the calories they consume. Overweight people, who are less active, store the unburned calories in the body as fat.

Based on the results of these studies, most overweight people can lose weight simply by maintaining their calorie intake and increasing their activity. For the severely obese, the studies indicate that excess weight is generally a result of too little activity and too much food. Following weight loss surgery, weight loss and maintenance will depend on a combination of eating a healthy, calorie appropriate, diet and being physically active.

THE BENEFITS OF EXERCISE...

Physicians use exercise as part of a comprehensive treatment plan for patients who have a variety of illnesses. Exercise is part of a rehabilitation program for heart patients. It is prescribed to help lower cholesterol, improve or abolish angina, and lower blood pressure. Exercise has been found to lower a diabetic's need for supplemental insulin. It has been of benefit in relieving muscle tension, headache, and sleep problems. Psychiatrists have noted that regular exercise leads to an improvement in the mood of patients who are depressed or anxious.

In addition to the many health benefits of exercise, there are a number of benefits of exercise for those wanting to achieve and maintain a lower body weight.

Benefits of Exercise for Weight Loss and Maintenance
1. Exercise increases metabolic rate. Exercise increases the rate at which calories are burned. This increase in rate continues for five to eight hours after the exercise session is finished. Because of the increase in the rate at which calories are burned, people who exercise lose weight up to 30 percent quicker than those who do not.
2. Exercise burns fat. During the first thirty to forty minutes of a workout, the body burns carbohydrate energy (glucose). After thirty to forty minutes, the body burns fat. Exercising for sixty minutes actually reduces fat tissue.
3. Exercise reduces appetite. Though the exact process is not understood, exercise does seem to affect the hunger-control center in the brain causing a person to feel less hungry. This may be because exercise helps the body get glucose to the cells more efficiently.
4. Exercise improves mood. Exercise encourages the secretion of endorphins into the body. Endorphins, also known as endogenous opiates, are

chemicals that occur naturally in the body. Their purpose is to relieve stress and promote a feeling of well-being. Since many people eat to relieve stress, the feeling of well-being serves to prevent overeating.

5. Exercise helps weight maintenance. Exercise increases muscle. Unlike fat tissue, muscle tissue is never at rest. It is constantly burning calories, even when a person is resting. The constant burning of calories contributes to maintenance of a lower weight.

6. Exercise helps prevent constipation. Along with good nutrition and adequate fluid intake, regular exercise helps to alleviate constipation, which is a common side-effect of dieting.

EXERCISING TO BURN FAT AND MAINTAIN WEIGHT LOSS...

Once a person commits to regular exercise for weight loss and maintenance, it becomes important to determine what kind of exercise is best. Most fitness experts agree that the best exercise for burning fat and maintaining weight loss is aerobic exercise.

Aerobic exercise is any physical activity done at a steady pace. While studies suggest that aerobic exercise—in addition to reduced calorie intake—may only slightly increase weight loss, it appears essential for weight maintenance. Good aerobic exercises for the severely obese are walking, biking, swimming, and low-impact calisthenics and dancing. Current research-based recommendations for the overweight or obese are an accumulation of 60 to 90 minutes (beyond any activity involved in daily living) of aerobic exercise done a minimum of five days a week.

Many weight loss surgery patients have not engaged in regular exercise for some time. Because of this, many physicians and physical therapists or trainers suggest a patient move into exercise slowly and carefully. For example, a patient might begin to exercise by walking for five minutes daily and, as able, add five minutes gradually to increase the aerobic exercise time to 60 to 90 minutes daily at least five days a week.

Building muscle or lean body tissue is important to the weight loss surgery patient for the two reasons already presented. Muscle tissue burns calories more efficiently than fat tissue and it burns calories more constantly than fat tissue. There is a third important reason for the weight loss surgery patient to develop muscle. As a patient loses weight, fat tissue turns to flabby tissue. Good muscle development or tone will help to reduce the appearance of flab.

Exercising To Build Muscle...

To develop muscle tissue, calisthenics or weight training exercises must be added to the aerobic routine. Once a patient has fully recovered from surgery and is walking—or doing another aerobic activity—25 minutes at a time, they might add 5 minutes of calisthenics to their workout. Once they have progressed to doing 30 to 40 minutes of aerobic activity, they might add 15 to 20 minutes of calisthenics or weight training to their workout.

GETTING THE MOST FROM AN EXERCISE WORKOUT...

Duration and frequency are the key elements of exercise following weight loss surgery. But exercise takes time and effort. Because of this, some patients will want to get the greatest possible gain for the time and energy they expend. Dr. Sharon Sneed, a registered dietitian and co-author of the book *Love Hunger,* recommends that her patients exercise at a level that allows them to talk between heavier breaths while exercising. This intensity is usually between 65 and 85% of maximum heart rate.

Taking your pulse is the best way to determine the heart rate level. The pulse can be taken at the carotid arteries located on either side of the Adam's Apple. The pulse can also be taken at the wrist.

To take the pulse at the wrist, place the second and third fingers of one hand on the opposite wrist just under the crease. Count the number of times the heart beats during sixty seconds while sitting quietly. This is the resting heart rate and is usually between seventy and eighty beats per minute. To find the optimal heart rate range for exercise, do the following:

Finding the Optimal Exercise Heart Rate Range

1. Subtract your age from two hundred twenty to find your maximum heart rate. *Example*: Two hundred twenty minus the age of forty equals a maximum heart rate of one hundred eighty.
2. Multiply your maximum heart rate by 0.65 and then by 0.85 to find the best exercise heart beat range. *Example*: 0.65 multiplied by 180 is 111; 0.85 multiplied by 180 is 153.
3. For a maximum workout, don't let the pulse drop below the low number or go above the high number. *Example*: A forty year old person must not let the pulse drop below 111 or go above 153 during an aerobic workout. The pulse should be taken two to three times during an exercise period.

PROTECTING THE BODY DURING EXERCISE...

Earlier we discussed what happens when people do too much exercise too quickly. They experience pain. They can damage muscles and tendons. To avoid these possibilities, it is important to exercise wisely by starting an exercise program at a low level of duration and intensity and gradually increasing the duration and intensity of activity as the body adapts. Three additional factors are also important.

First, be sure to wear comfortable clothing that is appropriate for the activity. If walking, wear a good pair of shoes that support and cushion the feet well. If walking outside, consider the type of terrain and the weather. Walking uphill or on uneven ground is harder than walking on flat, smooth ground. Wear cool clothing if it is warm. If it is cool, wear several light layers of clothing. Layers can be removed as the body heats up during exercise. Avoid exercising when it is hot. Keep hydrated by drinking plenty of water.

Second, prepare the muscles and tendons for activity by stretching. Stretch for five minutes before and five minutes after a workout. Third, start an exercise session slowly and gradually build up to the maximum level of intensity. Toward the end of an aerobic session, gradually slow down the intensity of exercise instead of just stopping suddenly.

It is human nature to move toward those things that we enjoy and move away from those things that we do not. When selecting an exercise, it is vitally important that a person choose one that they will enjoy. If it is not enjoyable, then it will not be done.

To choose an exercise, patients should think about what they like to do. If a woman likes to dance, then an exercise that involves dancing might be best. She could do tap, square, or ballroom dancing. She might try an aerobic dance class. If a couple likes the out of doors, they might try walking, hiking, or biking. If a man likes competitive sports, he might try racquetball or handball.

Another part of making exercise enjoyable is doing it with others. If you want or need the help of another person, find an exercise partner. Together you might walk during a lunch break or meet at a class several evenings each week. If you need an authority figure to hold you accountable and keep you going when it gets tough, you might work out with a personal exercise trainer. The expense of a trainer might be shared with an exercise partner.

Above all, it is important to choose an exercise program that will fit into your lifestyle. If you have small children, it may be impossible to get away for a class. You might, however, walk for an hour when your spouse comes home and can watch the children. If you have an irregular schedule, you might choose a low-impact aerobics video or purchase a treadmill so you can exercise at home whenever it fits into your schedule.

Exercise can also be made enjoyable by charting progress. Make a specific goal and plan a reward for when the goal is accomplished. A goal might be to walk two miles three times a week. When done, a reward should be given. If you set an exercise goal, you should be sure it can be accomplished in a short amount of time. If the goal is too long-range, the reward may be too far off for it to provide motivation. Remember, food is not a reward.

Choosing an Exercise...

Up to this point we have been discussing programmed exercise. Another beneficial form of exercise is integrated exercise. Integrated exercise includes anything we do to move our body, from making our bed, to walking up a flight of stairs, to pulling a few weeds in the garden.

A person who weighs 175 pounds can burn as many as two hundred eighty calories by walking up and down a flight of stairs several times a day! We all have many opportunities to engage in integrated exercise every day. To promote weight loss and maintenance, we should take every opportunity we can to move our bodies.

EXERCISE: JUST DO IT!

For the weight loss surgery patient, the most important thing to remember about exercise is this:

If you really want to lose weight and keep it off...
you've got to do as the Nike commercial says
and JUST DO IT!

The most successful patients are those who do. Many multidisciplinary weight loss surgery programs include a physical therapist on the team to help patients develop a personalized exercise program to maximize weight loss. If a physical therapist is available to you, seek and follow their advice.

Exercising for Weight Loss and Maintenance

98

T.C.

There are those who think just because you are overweight you are Fat and Lazy. I am here to say that I worked very hard at being fat. In fact, it was only after I had vertical stapled gastroplasty that I realized the effort it took to maintain my weight.

To be fat, I had to plan my day around fast food restaurants and donut shops. I needed to go to the bank regularly to insure I had enough money to stop at any and all fast food drive-thru windows. I had to find places to dump the evidence (empty food containers) before I returned home. It could take me up to two hours in the morning to find clothes in my closet to hide my weight from myself and everyone else. My clothes had to be washed a day in advance because I dare not put anything in the dryer. I made private shopping trips to the Large Women's clothing store and turned the shopping bags inside out so no one would know where I bought my clothes. I made sure to eat 80 percent of my food intake for the day before my spouse got home. I avoided seeing friends and family because I couldn't remember how much I weighed the last time I had seen them. Besides, food was my best friend. I would not go anywhere that I would have to exert any energy or do any physical activity. I wouldn't wear a bathing suit or shorts. I would look forward to the times I could just be alone and eat and eat and eat. I couldn't pos-

sibly have the time or the energy, God forbid, to change my lifestyle or to diet and exercise.

The point I want to make is it actually takes less time to keep yourself healthy. Or else, since gastroplasty, someone has added more hours to my day. I feel great and look younger. Eating food has become something I do three times a day, not all day. I can trust myself at home with sweets. I have so many things to occupy my time that have nothing to do with eating. I enjoy seeing friends for the sake of good conversation or gossip, not for any excuse to overeat. I can go shopping in a mall and shop at all the stores. It amazes me how much I can get done in an average day. I can now choose to do nothing all day instead of assuming there is nothing I can do.

It took gastroplasty for me to be able to balance my life! ∾

CHAPTER SEVEN

Attitudes for Weight Loss and Maintenance

Ever since human beings developed the ability to speak, we have been telling stories. Through our story telling we pass down our history from one generation to another, we attempt to explain the mysteries of life, and we try to teach the values and attitudes that we believe are important to successful living.

One story that tells about an attitude needed to successfully accomplish a goal is *The Little Engine That Could*. It is a story we usually tell to small children. But its meaning has value to people of all ages.

You probably remember this story. It's about a little engine that worked in a busy train yard doing whatever small moving jobs needed to be done. In the train yard were many engines bigger than he was. The small engine looked up to the bigger engines admiring them for their strength and their endurance in pulling heavily loaded cars over long distances.

One day there was an emergency and a trainload of supplies needed to be transported as quickly as possible. The job would be hazardous because the load had to be pulled up and over a very steep, high mountain. This was a job for the biggest, strongest engine in the yard.

As the story goes, the biggest engine set out on this task. He knew his task was a difficult one. As he approached the high mountain, he began to think to himself, "This is too hard. I can't make it!" And he couldn't. The big engine pulled his load back to the train yard reporting that the job was too difficult to be done. Because the need was urgent, other big engines tried. Like the biggest engine they thought the job was too tough to be done. They all returned to the train yard having failed to accomplish the goal.

The little engine wanted to try. The big engines scoffed at him and his arrogance. How could such a little engine accomplish a task that the big engines couldn't do? But the situation was desperate. The load had to be transported. The station master decided to let the little engine give it a try.

Indeed, the task was very hard and the little engine struggled with the weight of the loaded cars. When he saw the mountain in front of him he called upon all his strength. As he inched toward the steep slope he kept thinking to himself over and over, "This is hard, but I think I can, I think I can, I think I can." And he did!

The moral of this story is straight-forward and clear. If you believe in your ability to overcome the obstacles between you and your goal, you can do it, no matter how hard it may be!

Weight loss surgeries are valuable tools that will help you lose weight and keep it off permanently. But the road to achieving your goal weight will have obstacles to be overcome. These obstacles may make it difficult for you to protect your surgical procedure, make nutritious food choices and engage in regular exercise. Not doing these things may sabotage your success. Like the little engine, you will need positive attitudes that will give you the courage, determination, and perseverance to overcome the obstacles that are on the road to your goal.

In this chapter, we will discuss the kinds of obstacles you might encounter on your road to a healthy body weight. We will discuss the negative attitudes that will keep you from overcoming these obstacles. Finally we will discuss the positive attitudes needed to successfully achieve your goal.

Most people who have weight loss surgery look forward to all the wonderful things they want to happen to them when they have reached their goal weight. They dream about buying fashionable clothes in a regular department store or boutique. No more going to the specialty shops for "larger sizes." They envision feeling comfortable with themselves and anticipate increased social activity. No more sitting home being lonely and bored. They think about participating in sports, getting a better job, improvement in their health, continuing their education, an enriched marriage, having a child, and much more. They think about doing all the things they haven't done because of their excess weight.

What people don't think about is the long journey from where they are at the time of surgery to where they want to be when they reach their goal weight. During the presurgical process patients should be informed that they may have some difficult adjustments to make following surgery. No matter how informed they may be, most patients feel there is an element of "magic" in the surgical procedure. Magically, they will recover from the surgery, make the necessary lifestyle adjustments, and live a new life. It is a rude awakening when they run into an obstacle on the road to their goal weight.

It is important to know that every patient will encounter obstacles on the road to a healthier body weight. Almost every patient will face some obstacles; other obstacles will present themselves to some patients but not to others. As we identify these obstacles, it is also important to know that they can be overcome. We begin our discussion of obstacles with those that almost every patient will encounter.

Shortly after surgery, all patients become aware that they have lost their freedom of choice when it comes to food. As discussed, the surgical procedures reduce the amount of food that may be eaten and it is necessary to follow a specific nutritional plan.

Before surgery most patients are used to eating as much of whatever they want to eat whenever they want to eat it. It can be emotionally painful to experience a restriction in the amount of and kind of food that may be eaten. The first obstacle most patients face is how they will deal with this emotional pain. The best way to overcome the emotional pain is to go through a grieving process.

Grief is something we associate with death. But grief may be a part of other losses or life changes, too. The more emotional pain you feel about the loss of the freedom to eat, the more grieving you may do.

Patients who refuse to resolve the loss by grieving often "cheat" in their food intake. They attempt to stuff the stomach pouch with more food than it can hold. Or they may eat food that the healing pouch is not ready to process. Those who engage in these behaviors may experience chronic vomiting.

Every day we receive many signals to eat that are completely unrelated to the nutritional needs of our bodies. These eating signals are called triggers. A time of day may be a trigger. It is noon and we want to have lunch, hungry or not. Activities can be triggers. At the movies we want popcorn; at a ball game we want a hot dog. Feelings can also be triggers. When we are angry we may want to eat crunchy junk food such as chips. When we are sad we may want to eat smooth comfort food like ice cream. Whatever the time, activity or feeling, triggers lead to emotional cravings. An emotional craving is an intense desire to eat a certain food whether we are hungry or not.

Controlling emotional cravings is the second common obstacle patients must overcome. Eating in response to an emotional craving may sabotage weight loss and maintenance. This is because foods that are craved are usually very high in fat and total calories. They generally have little nutritional value and digest quickly, leaving your stomach pouch empty. An empty pouch provides you with the opportunity to eat more food than your body needs. Weight loss is stopped or weight regain occurs.

A third common obstacle that may be experienced is a weight plateau. The number of pounds and inches lost following weight loss surgery may be rapid. This is especially true during the first six weeks after surgery when food intake is most limited. Sooner or later, however, the rate at which pounds and inches are lost will slow down.

During weight loss there may be times when the rate of pounds and inches lost will stop completely. This is called a plateau. A plateau is a resting period during which the body adjusts to the chemical and biological changes it is undergoing. Following a regular nutritional and exercise routine during the plateau is usually enough to encourage weight loss to begin again within a few weeks.

When a plateau occurs it is very important to overcome this obstacle by continuing the regular routine. If a plateau continues for longer than a few weeks, an adjustment in calorie intake and/or exercise may be required. Adjustments include decreasing the total calories eaten each day and increasing the length of exercise sessions. During a plateau it is not unusual to feel discouraged or depressed. These feelings should be processed so they do not lead to increased eating which may lengthen the plateau or lead to weight regain.

In addition to these obstacles which may be experienced by almost every patient, there are other obstacles some may encounter. Among these are compulsive overeating in response to stress or to stuff down uncomfortable feelings. Also included is overeating due to emotional pain from hurtful relationships. If a patient is to achieve their goal weight, they must learn effective coping and problem solving skills. They must learn how to process their feelings. They must learn to recover from the pain of hurtful relationships. And they must learn to behave self-responsibly.

A special obstacle to weight loss and maintenance confronts only a few patients. This is the obstacle of chronic illness, either physical or mental. While some physical and mental disorders improve with weight loss, others do not. If a physical or mental illness cannot be improved with weight loss, it is vitally important that a patient get whatever assistance is necessary to manage the illness and keep it from unduly sabotaging their weight loss and maintenance program. Members of the support team may assist in the development of a special treatment program for patients with special mental or physical needs. Referral to additional treatment professionals or facilities may also be provided.

ATTITUDES THAT DISCOURAGE WEIGHT LOSS AND MAINTENANCE...

Almost every waking minute we engage in self-talk. Self-talk is the dialogue we have within ourselves through our thoughts. We use this internal thought dialogue to help us describe and interpret what goes on around us. If our self-talk is based on reality, our behavior and feelings are also based on reality and we function appropriately. If our self-talk is distorted, irrational or untrue, our behavior and feelings are inappropriate, as well.

Very few of us engage in reality based self-talk all the time. Identifying the negative ways we talk to ourselves and replacing them with more positive thought patterns will help us live more effectively. Psychologist Albert Ellis studied the ways we talk to ourselves and identified 21 irrational thought patterns that are the most disruptive to our functioning. Several are especially harmful to weight loss and maintenance. We will discuss six.

The first irrational self-talk pattern is, **"I am helpless and have no control over what happens in my life."** When you say this to yourself you become a victim. Your success or failure depends on what something or someone outside of you allows. You see the obstacles you encounter on the road to your goal weight as signs that you will fail. Feeling doomed to failure, you may engage in self-defeating behaviors such as eating too many high fat foods to the point that a leak or rupture occurs.

A second irrational thought pattern is, **"I must be unfailingly competent or perfect in all that I attempt to do."** When you agree with this irrational thought, you believe that you are either good or bad. To be good you should always follow your nutritional and exercise program to the letter. Any deviation means you are bad and do not deserve to succeed. To make a mistake is to be a mistake. With your first mistake you conclude that you might as well not even try to reach your goal.

The third irrational thought pattern is, **"I should not feel pain. If I am supposed to have something, it should come to me with little effort."** This is the irrational belief of the spoiled child. When you subscribe to this distorted thought, you believe that life should be easy and effortless. If an obstacle presents itself, you are quickly discouraged and give up the goal. You may blame others for putting the obstacle in your way or pretend that you really didn't want to reach the goal anyway!

A fourth pattern of distorted self-talk is, **"It is wrong to be selfish."** To successfully lose weight and maintain your goal, you must engage in good self-care. You must be able to attend to your special dietary needs and you must take time for exercise. These activities may require that your relationships and schedule undergo some adjustment. If you believe it is selfish to take care of yourself or to inconvenience others, you won't make the needed adjustments. Instead you will sacrifice your health and your happiness so as not to upset others.

A fifth untrue pattern of internal dialogue is, **"It is better to ignore the problems of living than to face them."** This belief, more than any other, leads to compulsive eating. When you believe that problems should be ignored rather than solved, you experience a constant nervous tension within you. Binge eating or constant snacking is one way people try to cope with this nervous energy. While you won't be able to binge on large amounts of food following one of the restrictive or combined restrictive/malaborptive procedures, you may be able to snack on high fat, high calorie foods that sabotage your weight loss.

The sixth and final pattern of irrational self-talk we will discuss is, **"The past determines the present."** Before having weight loss surgery, you probably lost and regained weight many, many times. Because of this pattern, you may feel that no weight loss program will work for you. The belief that you are destined to be fat may discourage you from making the lifestyle changes necessary for successful weight loss and maintenance.

ATTITUDES FOR SUCCESSFUL WEIGHT LOSS AND MAINTENANCE...

Portia Nelson wrote a poem that is used in many recovery groups, reprinted here on the next page.

Perhaps patterns of irrational self-talk have sabotaged all your past attempts to achieve and maintain a healthier body weight. They could continue to sabotage your goal even with the help of weight loss surgery. As Portia Nelson so beautifully illustrates in her poem, your patterns of thought and behavior can be changed so that you can have a healthier body and a happier life. You don't have to be falling into that deep hole of weight loss and regain time and time again. But you must work to change your irrational self-talk into more supportive, reality based attitudes. In the paragraphs below, the irrational self-talk patterns are reframed into rational thought patterns. As you integrate them into your life and let them guide your behavior, these

Attitudes That
Discourage
Weight
Loss and
Maintenance...

Autobiography in Five Short Chapters

I.
I walk down the street.
There is a deep hole in the sidewalk.
I fall in.
I am lost.
I am helpless.
It isn't my fault.
It takes forever to find a way out.

II.
I walk down the same street.
There is a deep hole in the sidewalk.
I pretend I don't see it.
I fall in again.
I can't believe I am in the same place,
but it isn't my fault.
It still takes a long time to get out.

III.
I walk down the same street.
There is a deep hole in the sidewalk.
I see it is there.
I still fall in… it's a habit.
My eyes are open.
I know where I am.
It is my fault.
I get out immediately.

IV.
I walk down the same street.
There is a deep hole in the sidewalk.
I walk around it.

V.
I walk down another street.

attitudes will help you reach and maintain your goal weight. Read through these six attitudes daily until you have integrated them into your life. You might also write them on sticky notes or cards and post them around the house to help you keep them in mind.

SIX ATTITUDES FOR SUCCESS!

"**Although I may not have total control over what happens in my life, I can always control myself and how I respond to what happens.**" This attitude will empower you. No matter what life brings to you, you can control yourself. You can choose to exercise instead of eat in response to a craving. You can choose to be proactive (instead of reactive) by finding effective ways to resolve or cope with whatever problems life brings to you.

"**While I will try to do my best, I will accept that I will sometimes fail to achieve my best.**" This attitude frees you to be human. It allows you to try, make mistakes, and try again. Your value as a person is not in question. You are not either good or bad. You are just a normal human being who learns and makes progress toward a goal through the process of trial and error. If you eat more calories one day than your nutritional program recommends, you eat fewer calories the next day. If you miss a day of exercise, you may choose to lengthen future exercise sessions by a few minutes until you make up the time.

"**Sometimes life is difficult and painful. If I want to be successful in life, I must persevere in spite of the difficulty and the pain.**" Psychiatrist M. Scott Peck, in his book, The Road Less Traveled, reminds us that life has been, is, and always will be difficult. He teaches that the way to cope with the difficulty is to be disciplined. You are disciplined when you do the things you know are good for you in spite of how difficult it is to do them. To cope with the pain of life, Dr. Peck urges you to treat yourself with love. You are loving when you care for and nurture yourself through your pain. If you accept that there will be obstacles along your road to successful weight loss, they won't surprise you. Instead you will find ways to encourage and nurture yourself through the difficult, sometimes painful process.

"It is good to be self-responsible." To be self-responsible is to attend to your own needs as well as you attend to the needs of the important others in your life. In support of a healthier body weight, you are self-responsible when you eat meals that provide for the nutritional needs of your body. Being self-responsible also means you take time for exercise and to participate in programs that support your health and personal well-being. It is also true that you are better equipped to attend to the needs of others when you take good care of yourself.

"I am committed to face and resolve the problems of living." Problems and the stress they cause do not go away just because you ignore them. In fact, the more you try to avoid your problems, the bigger they become. This attitude urges you to learn effective problem-solving skills. With these skills, you can solve your problems as quickly and effectively as possible. With your problems solved, you will feel calm and relaxed and have no need for nervous eating.

"My success depends upon my choices and my behavior in the present." Human beings have a remarkable capacity for change. You don't have to continue making poor choices and engaging in self-defeating behavior just because you have done so in the past. Begin today to replace old patterns of thinking and behavior that don't work, with new ones that do. If you do, successful weight loss and maintenance will be much easier!

Kathy

It seems that society is educated about drug and alcohol addiction to a greater extent than it is about food addiction. The same basic principles apply to those of us who use food as a drug. Yet fat people are still the brunt of jokes. I wish that average weight people understood why overweight people continue to overeat. Perhaps the jokes and ridicule would decrease.

It's not that fat people are lazy, stupid, unaware of their weight problems, or lacking in will power. We do not consciously choose to be obese. We are undeserving of the comments and misevaluations made at our expense. Drug addicts and alcoholics can hide their addictions from others when they want to. Fat people show their problem to the world 24 hours a day.

I binge on high fat foods for several reasons. Eating soothes me. It brings me comfort. It takes me away from my problems. Of course, I don't really solve my problems or escape them when I overeat. I just put off facing them. Being fat allows me to believe that weight is my problem rather than being a symptom of my problem. I can focus on fat and continue to hide from whatever deep, dark secret or evil problem is lurking within. I can distract myself from the reality of my life's disappointments. In some strange way it is easier to hide in food, and present myself to the world in a fat body, than it is to admit that I have many disappointments in my life. It is

*too much work, and too painful to dig through my past and
work toward recovery. While being fat is painful, these other
issues are more painful.*

*Having gastroplasty and losing 95 pounds forced me to hit
a wall of reality. I did not realize how much fear and pain
I would encounter when the pounds came off. Gastroplasty
has helped me in some ways. But I have not yet made a real
commitment to tackle the issues in my life that I need to in
order to recover. When I do, when I finally decide it is worth
going through the pain, I am sure gastroplasty will help me
take off the pounds I have regained and the additional forty
I want to lose.*

*For me gastroplasty was and is a tool. It is not the magic
wand I had hoped for. But it has enabled me to start on a difficult, long path. One that leads over a huge mountain. I hope
I can stay on the path and climb over that mountain.* ⬥

CHAPTER EIGHT

Relationships, Weight Loss and Maintenance

In 1965, Elaine, a woman in her mid-thirties, made an appointment to begin psychotherapy with marital therapist Richard B. Stuart. Although she believed she was a good wife and mother and a competent worker, Elaine felt like she was a total failure. She felt this way because she had failed to accomplish one very important personal goal. She had failed to achieve and maintain an average body weight.

Elaine was sixty pounds overweight. In describing her diet history to Richard, Elaine reported that she usually started five diets a year. With the best of her efforts, she lost about ten pounds. Then she regained those ten pounds as quickly as she had lost them. And with each diet, she added a few more pounds and lost more of her self-esteem.

Elaine told Richard she had tried psychotherapy before. Although the treatment had helped her gain insight into the problems that contributed to her weight, it had not helped her lose weight. Elaine kept getting bigger and bigger. With each pound she gained, she became more preoccupied with her weight. Elaine was desperate.

Richard didn't know how he could help. Elaine had already tried the most respected diets and forms of psychotherapy with no results. But Richard saw how desperate she was. He agreed to try to help Elaine if she was willing to experiment. Through long hours of research Richard developed a behavior modification program that did help Elaine. She lost 45 pounds in 52 weeks.

Elaine was so delighted that she referred overweight friends to Richard. With his behavior modification techniques these friends started to lose weight, too. Richard's practice grew to be made up almost exclusively of overweight women and he eventually started working with Weight Watchers International.

As successful as he was, Richard noticed that there was a segment of the overweight population with whom even he had little or no success. In association with Barbara Jacobson, Richard began a study of these overweight women to try to understand why his program failed and to discover what might work. Together Richard and Barbara designed and published two questionnaires. Fifteen thousand women responded to the first questionnaire and nine thousand women responded to the second. Along with the completed questionnaires many women sent long, detailed letters about their lives and failed attempts to lose weight.

Through the responses of these women, Richard and Barbara made an important discovery. For many women being overweight played an important role in keeping their marital relationships stable. Whenever they started to lose weight, their marriages became problematic. When they gained weight, those problems disappeared. For these women, losing weight meant having to cope with a strained marriage or to risk losing their marriage altogether.

Poet John Donne wrote, "No man is an island, entire unto itself." Each of us is involved in a relationship network that includes the members of the family into which we were born and the members of the family we create through marriage or other forms of commitment. It also includes close friends and those with whom we associate in a variety of work, educational and social situations. All these relationships have some power to influence and shape our lives. At best, our relationships sustain, support, and enrich our lives. At their worst, they hurt, sabotage, and diminish us.

As discussed before, the decision to lose weight with the aid of weight loss surgery is a very personal one. It is only when you have decided for yourself that it is important to achieve a healthy body weight that you will make the lifestyle changes necessary to do it. But you won't be able to go it alone. You will need help from family and friends. In this chapter we will discuss how relationships can help or hinder your efforts toward your goal weight.

GOOD RELATIONSHIPS SUPPORT HEALTH…

Humans are complex beings with a number of important needs. According to psychologist Abraham Maslow, our needs fit into five basic categories.

Basic Human Needs
- **Physiological Needs**: Our need for enough oxygen, water, food, shelter and rest to insure our survival.
- **Safety Needs**: Our need to live in an environment that is reasonably consistent, orderly and fair.
- **Belonging Needs**: Our need to give and receive care, love and affection.
- **Esteem Needs**: Our need to feel personally adequate, competent, confident, independent, and free. Our need to know that others recognize, appreciate, and respect us.
- **Self-Actualization Needs**: Our need to continually learn, grow and develop our potential. Our need to do things that contribute to the development of those people with whom we relate and to those organizations to which we belong.

Maslow suggests that our health and well-being depends upon how well these needs are met. While meeting these needs requires individual responsibility and effort, we also benefit from the support and help of family and friends.

Good relationships are those that encourage us and help us adequately meet all of our needs. Certainly good relationships provide for the satisfaction

Good Relationships Support Health…

of our physiological needs. But our physiological needs are not provided for at the expense or exclusion of any other need. In good relationships we also want to talk and play. We want to share our joy, sorrow, hopes and dreams. We want to encourage and challenge each other to be and do our best. We want to nourish each other by the quality of our interaction as much as by the food we eat. Good relationships promote our physical, emotional, intellectual, social and spiritual health and well-being.

RELATIONSHIPS THAT CAN MAKE US FAT...

In an ideal world all of our relationships would be as helpful and supportive as we would like them to be... all of our needs would be perfectly satisfied. But we don't live in an ideal world. Rarely are our relationships as nurturing as we wish them to be. And rarely are our needs met completely. But that is okay. Our relationships only need to be good enough; our needs must only be met adequately. And for most of us our relationships are good enough and our needs are adequately met.

But some relationships are not good enough. Instead, they are deficient in one or more ways. Sometimes our needs are not met because of our choices and behaviors in our relationships. We may also allow the choices and behaviors of others to interfere with the meeting of our needs. Whoever is responsible, the neglect or suppression of our needs may lead to varying kinds of physical, emotional, intellectual, social and spiritual illness. One of these illnesses is severe obesity.

Psychiatrist David Viscott had some valuable things to say about the effect of our choices and behaviors within relationships. According to Dr. Viscott, we best meet our needs and support others to meet their needs when we are emotionally free. In his book, *Emotionally Free*, he describes what this means as...

> "...the natural feeling state of the evolved mature person. (Being emotionally free) constitutes your ability to react honestly to events in the present... It reflects your capacity to act in your own best interest without seeking approval or permission...

Because emotional freedom is born of self-acceptance, when you are emotionally free you have nothing to prove. You are also aware of a sense of commonality with other people so that when you act freely you do not compromise the rights of others, but allow them to be free as well."

Most of us are not fully evolved and mature; therefore, we are not emotionally free. Instead we carry around emotional baggage that burdens us. This emotional baggage is the result of unresolved disappointments and hurtful experiences from the past and/or worrisome fears and concerns for the future. Depending on the nature of the emotional baggage and our own personality, we behave in one of three relationship styles. These relationship styles are dependent, controlling, or competitive. All three styles have their strengths and their weaknesses. The strengths enable us to behave in ways that meet our own needs and to encourage others to meet their needs, as well. The weaknesses lead to behaviors that sabotage ourselves and others.

THE THREE RELATIONSHIP STYLES

A person may be described as dependent when their primary orientation is having and caring for relationships. The strengths of a dependent person are loyalty, sincerity, warmth, affection, and caring. At their best, a dependent person will genuinely support and nurture themselves as well as others. They want for themselves and others an opportunity to experience life fully and to be all that they can be. The weaknesses of a dependent person include being clingy, insecure, jealous, and fearful of being rejected or alone. At their worst, a dependent person will overly protect themselves. They will cling to another in a way that will make it impossible for that person to meet their own needs.

The controlling person is one who is focused upon keeping things orderly. The strengths of a controlling person are the ability to be organized, responsible, and disciplined. Because they can anticipate problems, they make life simpler for themselves and others. The weaknesses of a controlling person include being petty, vindictive, and punitive. They can treat themselves and others in hurtful ways when their expectations are not met.

The competitive person is basically concerned with accomplishing goals and being rewarded. At their best, a competitive person is a doer. They set a goal and work to meet it. At their worst, a competitive person can be self-centered, childish, and ruthless. They pursue what they want without any consideration of others.

When you and those with whom you relate are functioning from your strengths, your relationships will be good enough. You will seek to provide one another with support, encouragement, and nurture. You will negotiate the satisfaction of needs and solve problems in ways that are mutually rewarding and satisfying. You will genuinely celebrate one another's accomplishments and successes.

If you and those close to you relate to each other from a position of weakness, your relationships will be, to some degree, dysfunctional. You will sabotage your own goals, or you will allow yourself to be sabotaged by others. Here are a few of the reasons people keep themselves fat or why others try to keep them fat.

Reasons For Self-Sabotage
- "I'm afraid I won't be able to take care of myself on my own. If I appear helpless and needy (severely obese), someone will take care of me. If I appear too capable, I might have to face life alone."
- "I'm afraid that I will do something bad if I am thinner. I'm afraid I won't be able to control my behavior." (This is especially true of sexual behavior).
- "I'm afraid that others will expect more from me than I can do. If I stay fat, people won't expect me to achieve very much. I won't have to face the possibility of failing."
- "If I am fat, I won't be abused anymore."

Reasons for Others to Sabotage You
- "If my family member/friend is fat, they won't leave me. They won't feel that they can find a better family member/spouse/friend than I am."

- "If my family member/friend is fat, they will feel grateful to have me. I can control them. They will put up with my demands and bad behavior."
- "If my family member/friend is fat, I won't have to worry about them being better than I am. No matter what they can do well, their ability will always be hidden by their weight. I can always be the best."
- "If my family member/friend is fat, they will be too weak to keep me from abusing them."

Whether you choose to eat to the point of severe obesity or are encouraged to do so by another, the negative consequences to your health are profound. To improve your overall health through weight loss, you will need to improve the health of your dysfunctional relationships as well. But before you are ready to confront others, you must first face and stop your own self-defeating behavior. You can do this by learning to be your own best friend.

BEING YOUR OWN BEST FRIEND...

Take a moment to picture your best friend. See their face. Get in touch with how you feel about your friend. Think about the way you treat them. As you see your friend in your mind's eye, you probably see them as attractive. This attractiveness comes not so much from your friend's actual physical appearance as much as your experience of the quality of their character. To you they are pretty inside and out. Your feelings for your friend are warm and cozy. You always want the best for your friend and take delight in their achievement and success. You treat your best friend with respect and consideration. You are always there to support and encourage your friend through thick and thin. Even when they disappoint you or make you angry, you value them so much that you wouldn't think of mistreating them. You don't need your friend to be perfect. You accept their weaknesses as well as strengths.

Now consider how you treat yourself. Do you treat yourself the way you treat your best friend? If you are like most severely obese people, you probably don't. Instead, you may feel afraid of your needs. You may treat yourself with indifference, neglect, or outright hostility. This is not unusual. Many obese people feel like they will do something bad if they try to fulfill their

119

needs. They see themselves as misfits and failures and believe that they don't deserve to succeed. Some mistakenly believe that self-punishment will eventually motivate them to get serious about losing weight.

The best way to motivate yourself toward successful weight loss and maintenance is not through indifference, neglect, or punishment. It is through treating yourself in ways that are respectful, considerate, supportive and rewarding. Here are some suggestions for being your own best friend.

Being Your Own Best Friend

- Talk to yourself with kindness and respect. Refuse to call yourself any negative, critical or abusive names.
- Take good care of yourself. Consider your needs as important as the needs of those you care for and about.
- Live your life well. Add elegance, order, beauty, and joy to your everyday living experience.
- Be considerate of your feelings. Process your feelings by keeping a journal or by talking them through with a confidant.
- Support your efforts for change. Learn from and grow through your mistakes.
- Record and reward your progress. Celebrate each success no matter how small it may be.

You may have some things you would like to add to this list. Whatever you do, remember that you will only achieve and maintain a healthier body weight by relating to yourself in a friendly, supportive manner.

GETTING HELP FROM FAMILY AND FRIENDS...

Those who truly care about you want you to be healthy and happy. They are usually willing to do whatever they can to help you reach your goal weight. However, they don't always know what is best to do. If left to guess, they may do the wrong things. And you can't expect them to demonstrate their love for you by reading your mind. A better approach is to tell them exactly what you need. Tell them the type of supportive attitudes and behaviors that will be helpful to you. There are several that you may find beneficial.

Friends and family can help you by being understanding about just how challenging it is for you to achieve your goal weight and maintain it. You will need to educate them about what weight loss surgeries are and how they work. Like you, your friends and family need to accept that the procedures are not magic but valuable tools for successful weight loss and maintenance.

Once they understand what the procedures are and how they work, your friends and family can believe in your ability to be successful. Because they are close to you, they probably know of your previous attempts to lose weight that have failed. They need to talk and act as if this time you will be successful.

To practically support your weight loss your friends and family will need to make necessary environmental and behavioral changes. High-calorie, high-fat food will need to be removed from your environment. Healthy menus and foods will need to be planned and prepared. If eating out has been a frequent recreational activity, new ways of having fun together will need to be developed. Together you will need to identify dysfunctional behavior patterns and replace them with healthy ways of interacting.

The gift of time is another way friends and family can be of practical support. Taking over a household chore may provide you with much needed time to do weight loss activities such as exercising or attending support classes. The gift of companionship may also be helpful. Enjoying the company of a friend or family member during your exercise workout may be more motivational than having to do it alone.

Another valuable way of supporting you in your weight loss and maintenance program is by being flexible. Some of the changes you need family and friends to make may be difficult or inconvenient for them. You need them to be flexible enough to work through any challenge these changes may present.

One last thing that family and friends can do is celebrate your success. They can do this by complimenting you on how well you are doing and by giving you an occasional reward. It is very encouraging to have your effort and progress recognized and rewarded.

Getting Help from Family and Friends...

In addition to these helpful things that family and friends can do, there are two things they should never, ever do. First, friends and family should never try to police your behavior. You and only you are in charge of when and what you eat and when and how you exercise. It is not helpful if friends and family try to control or direct these activities. Second, friends and family should never test your resolve. They should never tempt you with foods or activities that could sabotage your success.

Is help from friends and family really all that important? The answer is a resounding yes! Dr. David R. Black, PH D, associate professor of health promotion at Purdue University studied the success rate of dieters. Dr. Black found that dieters with supportive partners lose significantly more weight and do better at keeping it off than dieters who go it alone.

OTHER SOURCES OF SUPPORT...

Family and friends do play a very important role in providing you with support. But there are times when you may need more support, or a different kind of support, than they can provide. You may also need help from a support group. Many weight loss surgery programs provide access to groups and professionals that can give you the extra support you need. These services are available in the community at large, as well.

Support groups such a Overeaters Anonymous, Overcomers Outreach, and Weight Watchers are available in almost every community. In selecting a support group, be sure that the group will accept and work with your special dietary needs. You will not be able to follow the standard dietary programs that some groups provide or require. Whether you participate in a group you find on your own or one sponsored by your surgical program, it is best to choose a group that provides you with these important services: Technical Support, Technical Challenge, Emotional Support, Emotional Challenge, and Shared Social Reality.

Five Important Support Group Services

- **Technical Support**: Giving you information needed to make wise decisions about nutrition, exercise, relationships and other lifestyle behaviors important for weight loss and maintenance.
- **Technical Challenge**: Encouraging you to learn and try new foods, activities, and behaviors.
- **Emotional Support**: Understanding and support as you face the difficult challenges involved in making the lifestyle changes necessary to weight loss and maintenance.
- **Emotional Challenge**: Encouragement to overcome any obstacles to making life-style change. Challenge to learn helpful ways of expressing your emotions and solving problems.
- **Shared Social Reality**: Letting you know you are "normal" in your feelings and behaviors. Letting you know you are not alone in the challenges you face in making the lifestyle changes needed following weight loss surgery.

Other Sources of Support...

In addition to group support, some people require individual psychotherapy following weight loss surgery. Individual psychotherapy is often beneficial to those who have been sexually abused or have experienced other abusive and/or dysfunctional relationships. It is estimated that up to 85 percent of those who are severely obese have had abusive and/or dysfunctional relationship experiences.

Individual psychotherapists include Psychiatrists, Psychologists, Marriage and Family Therapists, and Licensed Clinical Social Workers. Psychiatrists are a good choice if you require psychotropic medication as part of your treatment. For psychotherapy without medication, Psychologists, Marriage and Family therapists and Licensed Clinical Social Workers are good choices for helping you recover from or resolve issues of individual or relationship dysfunction.

As in choosing a support group, you should be sure that an individual psychotherapist is acquainted with weight loss surgical procedures or is willing to consult with your professional surgical and support team about the procedure and its lifestyle requirements. Be sure the psychotherapist is acquainted with the eating issues common to those who have experienced abuse and/or other kinds of relationship dysfunction. Also be sure that the psychotherapist will help you to find your own resolutions to the problems and challenges you face. In both a support group and in individual therapy, the focus should be on helping you reach your weight loss goal by resolving any individual or interpersonal issues that may interfere with this goal. Groups or individual therapy situations that focus upon the discussion of problems without moving toward the resolution of those problems are best avoided.

RELATIONSHIPS THAT ARE RESISTANT TO CHANGE...

Severe obesity is a complex problem involving many psychological and interpersonal issues. If you are to achieve and maintain a healthy body weight, you will need to resolve these issues. While you will always be in control of personal change, you may not be able to get those around you to make the changes necessary to your health and well-being. Because they are competitive, controlling, dependent, or engaged in their own self-destructive behavior, some friends and family members may resist positive change. They may continue to sabotage your success.

Sometimes friends, marital partners and family members need you to be just as understanding and supportive of their challenges in making change as you want them to be of yours. By being loving and supportive, you can strengthen and enrich your relationships so that they are better than ever. Marital or family therapy may help you to do this.

Unfortunately, no matter how understanding and supportive you are, those close to you may strongly resist any change. They may want you to remain fat so that they can feel comfortable. Should anyone have to sacrifice their health and well-being so that another person can feel comfortable? As painful as it may be, you may need to distance yourself from or give up the relationship in order to protect your health and well-being. Psychotherapy can help you determine if distancing from or leaving a relationship is your best alternative.

124

Successfully achieving and maintaining a healthy body weight will bring many changes to your life. The physical changes are the ones most weight loss surgery patients dream about. They dream about an end to all the aches and pains they feel due to severe obesity. They fantasize about walking into a department store or boutique to buy a "normal size" dress or shirt off the rack. They envision themselves doing all the things they couldn't do because they were too fat, such as riding a roller coaster, playing a sport, and much more.

As the health of your body improves, the quality of your relationships may improve, as well. First you may notice that you feel differently about yourself. Successfully losing weight and keeping it off may give you a new sense of self-confidence and self-esteem. You may feel like you want to be more and do more. Life may become a more exciting adventure.

A better relationship with yourself often brings opportunities for better relationships with others. As you enjoy yourself and life more fully, you can be much more fun to be around. Energy and enthusiasm for life is attractive to others. Old friendships can become closer. New friendships can be made. Family times can be more fun. And romantic relationships can begin or be renewed.

No one can promise you that all your relationship dreams will come true because you have a slimmer body. But many wonderful relationship opportunities may come your way. Let them enrich your life. A good relationship, with yourself and/or others, is more satisfying and less fattening than food.

Enjoying New and Renewed Relationships...

*I've been
there...*

Roy

I am a compulsive overeater and seven and one-half months ago I had gastric bypass surgery. At the time of surgery, I weighed 514 pounds. Even now, as I look at that monstrous number, I am embarrassed and ashamed of it. I have a hard time believing that my weight had gotten so high.

For most of my life, especially from my college years and beyond, my weight became untenable. I had tried all of the various weight loss programs around. On more than one occasion, I lost in excess of 100 pounds. Each time I put that weight back on and more. Two things were evident from this. First, none of the traditional weight loss methods are designed to deal with long term weight control, especially for those who are excessively overweight. Second, they tend to be run by women who do not understand their male clientele very well. Too many times I found myself in a program surrounded by women who were trying to lose fifteen pounds. It seemed ludicrous. I was able to do that in a week, if I wanted.

Once my weight reached 375 pounds, things in my life began to deteriorate. I could no longer participate in many activities I loved. I became visually obtrusive. Society is strange. Women are judged harshly for every pound they are overweight. Men often find their weight laughed off. To become socially unacceptable, a man has to carry a truly unhealthy amount of weight. I am 6 feet 4 inches tall. A comment I heard often was, "you carry a lot of weight well." I had reached a weight where

I've been there...

I did begin to experience social stigma. It only caused me to retreat more into food and denial.

I lived in denial for a couple of years. I knew Icontinued to put on weight. I lied to myself that it wasn't really that bad and that I could always go on a diet and take the weight off again. And, if I did, this time I would keep it off. It didn't work out that way. Fad diets could no longer produce the effects Idesired. I hated myself for not having the will power to succeed. I did what any normal compulsive overeater would do, I ate more just to relax and forget my weight and the pain it caused me.

I kept putting on weight. My weight began to affect my job performance and ultimately cost me my job. I no longer had energy to do anything. I suffered from such a severe case of sleep apnea that I would awake every 45 minutes throughout the night. I could not walk without a limp due to arthritis in both knees and severe pain in my back caused by the weight. I would fall asleep everywhere, even while I was driving. I became a social recluse hiding in food and planning my next meal. I would plan visits to the drive-throughs of fast food restaurants so no one would notice how much I was eating. I felt like I was in a living hell with no hope of ever getting out.

I had known about gastric surgery for some time, but never considered it to be an option for me. I felt as if I would be giving in or admitting failure if I had surgery for weight loss. The only reason I finally chose to have the operation was because it was either that or die. And I have to admit that, because I had no life to speak of and was terribly depressed, death seemed a comforting option.

After changing insurance providers once, the surgery was approved. Since having the surgery, I regret that I did not act sooner. I have lost 200 pounds and have not felt this good in years. My sleep apnea is gone; so is the pain in both my back and knees. For the most part, my depression is also gone. I am beginning to feel alive again. If I had not had gastric bypass, I know that by now I would be dead, or very close to being dead.

I still label myself a compulsive overeater. I will be for the rest of my life. This is a fact. The thing I have now is a tool that restricts my expression of this behavior. Though I still struggle with my psychological desire to eat compulsively, for the first time ever I have a tool to defeat this scourge. I am more incredibly thankful than words could ever express. ∾

I've been there...

CHAPTER NINE

Stress Management for Weight Loss and Maintenance

In the past twenty-plus years, I have had the opportunity to interview hundreds of candidates for weight loss surgery. During the interview most candidates acknowledge that they eat more food than they need to eat for the nourishment of their body. So, I ask each one if there are some times when they are more likely to overeat than others. Common answers to this question include…

"When I am upset."

"When I feel pressured."

"When I am alone and bored."

"At work (or home) when I have too much to do."

"When I am nervous."

"When I am angry."

"When I have to drive a long distance or in heavy traffic."

"When I need to relax."

Almost without exception, the answer involves overeating in response to stress.

Following weight loss surgery, many of these same people participate in my patient education and support group programs. Together we talk about the lifestyle changes they need to make in order to get maximum benefit from the surgical procedure. We share the excitement and joy they feel as their weight decreases. We work to overcome any obstacles they encounter on the road to their goal weight. Over and over we focus upon the fact that, even though weight loss surgeries are valuable tools, they are not magic. To achieve and maintain their goal weight will require them to continually make wise lifestyle choices.

Somewhere along the road to their goal weight, many people find themselves reverting to an old behavior. They eat in response to stress. Because of their surgical procedure, they cannot eat the quantity of food they ate previously when they were stressed. But the quality of the food they choose to eat when stressed is usually low in density and high in calories. As you may remember from earlier discussion, low density foods (chips, candy, ice cream) liquefy quickly and empty from the pouch faster than high density foods (meats, fruits and vegetables, cereals). Low density, high calorie foods raise your caloric intake above that required for weight loss or weight maintenance. Eating in response to stress may lead to a weight plateau or a regain of weight. For patients who have had a combined or mostly malabsorptive procedure, eating foods high in sugar or fat may lead to dumping or diarrhea.

If you have the habit of eating in response to stress but want to protect your weight loss, it is vitally important that you learn and practice effective techniques for stress management. In this chapter, we will discuss just what stress is and we will suggest some good stress management techniques.

WHAT STRESS IS...

Stress has been defined in many ways. A concise definition of stress is one given by Dr. Martha Davis and her co-authors in, *The Relaxation and Stress Reduction Workbook*. Dr. Davis says...

"Stress is any change that you must adjust to."

Stress can be things like getting fired, having an argument with someone, too many bills to pay for the amount of money you have, and finding your weight went up five pounds. All things we consider to be bad. But good things can also require change. Stress can be buying the house of your dreams, getting a job promotion and raise, falling in love, and finding that your weight went down five pounds. The negative things that require change we call distress; the positive things we call eustress. According to Dr. Davis, we experience stress from three sources: our environment, our body, and our thoughts.

All day, everyday, our environment presents us with the need to adjust. There are changes in the weather, noise levels, number of people with whom we interact, the amount of traffic on the freeway. There are changes in the number of things we have to do and the amount of time in which we have to do them. There are changes in our interpersonal demands and our work and home responsibilities. There are numerous threats to our physical and emotional security or self-esteem.

Our bodies present us with changes that must be made either slowly or rapidly. The natural process of growth and aging requires gradual change. Illness and accident require immediate change. The need for food and rest require adjustment. Environmental factors such as problems, demands, and dangers require the body to adjust.

The third source of stress is your thoughts. Your thoughts are how you interpret your experiences from the past and/or present and predict your experience in the future. Dwelling on some unpleasant experience in the past is stressful. Solving or not solving a problem in the present is stressful. Worrying about what might happen in the future is stressful.

Most often when we think of the stress placed upon us by the changing demands of our environment, body, and thoughts, we think of having too many things to which we must adjust. Many of us feel that the number of demands placed upon us each day is unreasonable. We live in a constant state of panic trying to do as many things as we can. While we are doing them we worry that we won't get them done before we run out of time, money, energy, or before new demands are added to our "to do" list.

But having too little to do can be as stressful as having too much to do. To be fulfilled, we need stimulation and challenge. When life is too predictable, routine and dull, it is stressful. While recreational distractions make life interesting for a while, sooner or later they also become uninspiring. Living life fully requires doing and accomplishing things that provide us with a sense of purpose. It means doing things that enrich our lives as well as the lives of others.

HOW WE RESPOND TO STRESS...

Physiologically we are designed to respond to stress in some predictable ways. Within us we have an automatic "flight or fight" response. This automatic response is triggered whenever we become aware of a need to adjust to a threat. As soon as we feel threatened in any way, we prepare to confront (fight) or escape (flight) the threat. Our pupils enlarge and our hearing becomes more acute; the better to see and hear our adversary. Our muscles tense; the better to strike out or run. Our heart and respiratory rate increases. Blood drains from our extremities and collects in our trunk and our head. The redistribution of blood and oxygen helps us think more clearly and act more quickly; the better to decide whether it is best to run or attack and then to act on that decision.

This flight or fight response was necessary for the survival of our ancient ancestors. When confronted with an adversary, like a saber-toothed tiger, these physiological changes enabled them to assess the situation quickly and prepare to fight or run like heck. Because this response helped them survive, through the process of natural selection it was passed down from generation to generation. Today this fight or flight response is an innate part of our biochemical makeup.

The kinds of threats we experience are different from those of our ancient ancestors. We don't have saber-toothed tigers with which to deal. But our complex lifestyle presents us with a variety of stressors. We cope with the challenge of getting to work on time, heavy freeway traffic, meeting deadlines, juggling hectic family schedules, and more. In fact, the amount of stress we deal with is many times greater than that of our predecessors. Our increased amount of stress presents us with a unique problem.

For our ancient ancestors, once a fight or flight was finished, the stress ended. All the physiological responses that took place to prepare the body for action reversed themselves. Physiologically they relaxed. For many of us today, once we have adapted to one stressor we are immediately confronted with another. Our bodies don't have time to relax. Instead, the body remains in a constant state of alert ready for flight or fight. Living in a constant state of alert contributes to physiological wear and tear, which may lead to a number of illnesses. Among these are hypertension, headache, ulcer, arthritis, colitis, diarrhea, asthma, cardiac arrhythmia, poor circulation, sexual problems, muscle tension and cancer. We can add severe obesity to this list.

Since the need to adapt to change is a fact of life, we will always experience stress. But we do have some important choices regarding stress that we can and need to make.

We can often choose the kind or amount of stress we experience.
We can choose how we respond to the stress we experience.
We can choose to take care of ourselves when we experience stress.

In order to do these things we must learn the art of self-responsibility. We must learn to be proactive in our response to stress. Finally, we must learn to take good care of ourselves when we are stressed (instead of eating).

THE IMPORTANCE OF SELF-RESPONSIBILITY...

As children we receive clear messages from our parents about how we should behave. One message most of us received was not to be selfish. We were told to share, to think of others first and that it is better to give than receive. To be selfish was to do what you wanted to do without regard for anyone else. To be selfish was to be bad.

Unfortunately, many people learned this message too well. They interpreted it to mean that any self-concern or self-interest was selfish. As adults they feel like they are doing something wrong anytime they consider their own wants and needs, any time they try to take control of their own lives. They often run themselves ragged trying to take care of the wants and needs of everyone else with little regard for their own well-being.

If you believe that you must respond to others without consideration of your own needs, you will lose control of your own life. You will experience chronic stress. Your sense of being out of control and feeling chronically stressed may have been what led you to eat to severe obesity. If you continue to eat in response to stress, you can sabotage your weight goal even following weight loss surgery.

Adults must sometimes unlearn things they were taught in childhood. Or at least they must restructure the childhood message to fit adulthood. For example, as a child you were probably taught not to cross the street alone or to hold someone's hand when you did cross the street. It is absolutely silly to think that, as an adult, you would not cross the street if alone or that you would reach out to take a stranger's hand before crossing! So we must restructure our childhood concept of what it is to be selfish. As an adult we must learn to balance our other-responsibility with self-responsibility. We must learn to act in our own self-interest to protect our physical and mental health from the negative aspects of stress.

What does it mean to be self-responsible? In their book, *Expressing Your Feelings*, psychiatrists Robert T. and Theresa L. Crenshaw define it as:

> *"Acting in your own best self-interest, having considered your wants and goals, the long-and short-term results of your actions and the possible effects of your actions on those you care about."*

If you truly want to reach your goal weight following weight loss surgery, you will need to take self-responsibility very seriously. Reaching your goal weight will require taking time to prepare nutritious meals and to eat slowly and carefully. It will require you to engage in regular exercise. It will require you to learn about and make all the lifestyle changes necessary to support your weight loss and maintenance. Finally, it will require that you overcome any obstacles you encounter on the road to weight loss.

Your environment will present you with many demands for change. Some of these will be beneficial to your weight goal and some will sabotage it. As a self-responsible person, you must assess each situation. Then you must say "yes" to those situations that support your wants and goals and "no" to the others. When you are self-responsible you have more power to direct your life than you may have realized. You can choose to say yes to change and adjustment or you can say no.

With regard to your weight loss goals you can...

Say Yes To

1. Things that simplify your life. You want to strike a balance between the time you spend working and taking care of others and relaxing and attending to your own needs. You won't be able to maintain a perfect balance at all times. But you can re-establish a balance as soon as you realize you are experiencing the stress of being out of balance.
2. Opportunities you can find for exercise, nutritious foods, adequate relaxation and rest.

You can...

Say No To

1. Things that complicate your life so that you have no time to take care of yourself. Demands will always come your way. Whenever possible, say no to those things that will overcommit you and leave you feeling out of control.
2. Situations that discourage exercise, healthy eating, sufficient relaxation and rest.

Contrary to what you may believe, the world will not fall apart if you say no to some of the demands placed upon you. Yes, someone may be miffed for a short time, but most of the time it won't be a catastrophe. By talking through the situation, you can negotiate a solution that is self-responsible and other-responsible.

The Importance of Self-Responsibility...

137

So take time to look at your life. Determine several needs and goals. Decide what you need to eliminate from your lifestyle (to say no to) so that you have the time, energy, and state of mind to add (to say yes to) those things that will help you accomplish your goals. Your goal of achieving and maintaining a healthy body weight should be a priority on that list! By making self-responsible choices about what you do, you will reach your goal weight and, in general, decrease the amount of stress in your life.

BEING PROACTIVE...

In addition to making choices about the kind and amount of stress we experience, we must also make choices about how we will respond to stress. In his book, *The 7 Habits of Highly Effective People*, Stephen R. Covey suggests that we generally respond to stress in one of two ways. Either we are proactive or we are reactive.

As we have discussed, all of us are presented with demands for change and adjustment. While we cannot choose what the demands might be, we can choose whether or not we will make the change or adjustment. We can also choose how we will respond to the demand.

When a stressor presents itself, our first response is usually emotional. Having emotional responses to people, places, and things is part of what makes us human. If the stressor is a change or adjustment to something we like, we have good feelings. If the stressor is something we don't like, we have bad feelings.

To be reactive is to let your feelings determine how you will behave in response to a stressor. If a stressor triggers anger, you may rant and rave and eat. If a stressor triggers hurt, you may sulk and eat. If a stressor triggers fear, you may behave as if you are a helpless victim and eat. Behavior that is triggered by an emotional response doesn't take care of the stressor. Sometimes it even makes the stress and our bad feelings about it worse. Likewise, eating doesn't resolve the stressor or our bad feelings. It just makes us fat.

To be proactive is to feel your feelings in response to the stressor but to also think and choose the most effective behavior needed to take care of the stressor. If a stressor triggers anger, you carefully choose behavior that will respond to the stressor and end your anger. If a stressor triggers hurt, you carefully choose behavior that will respond to the stressor and end your hurt. If a stressor triggers fear, you carefully choose behavior that will respond to the stressor and end your fear. Behavior that is based on thought and careful choice resolves the stressor and leaves us feeling emotionally free.

A way to determine if you are reactive or proactive is to look at where you focus your time and energy. Covey suggests that we all have a Circle of Concern. (*See figure 11*.) Our Circle of Concern contains a wide range of things with which we are mentally and emotionally involved. These things include our job, family, finances, weight, general health, the national debt, the possibility of natural disaster and much more.

As we look at the things within our Circle of Concern, it is clear that it contains some things that we can do something about and some things over which we have no control. The things we can do something about may be grouped within a smaller circle inside our Circle of Concern. This is our Circle of Influence. (*See figure 11*).

We are reactive when we spend more time and energy focused on the things within our Circle of Concern than on the things within our Circle of Influence. In other words, we spend more time and energy on things over which we have no control than we do on things we can do something about. When you focus on your Circle of Concern you often feel helpless and victimized. You blame others for your circumstances and want someone else to fix them. You neglect areas you could do something about. This increases your stress and your bad feelings about it and may lead you to eat.

When you focus on your Circle of Influence, your time and energy is spent on making good behavioral choices. These behavioral choices help you solve your problems and reduce your stress. As this happens, your feelings of self-confidence and self-control increase. Effective problem solving, self-confidence and self-control empower you to meet your needs and accomplish your goals. When you are empowered you eat when you are hungry, not when you are stressed.

Achieving and maintaining a healthy body weight following weight loss surgery is within your Circle of Influence. You can focus your time and energy on it by learning to think and choose effective behavior in response to

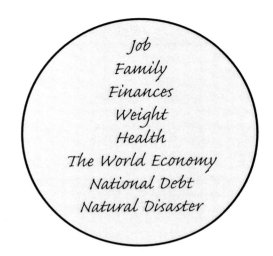

Job
Family
Finances
Weight
Health
The World Economy
National Debt
Natural Disaster

CIRCLE OF CONCERN

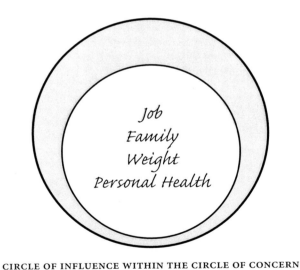

Job
Family
Weight
Personal Health

CIRCLE OF INFLUENCE WITHIN THE CIRCLE OF CONCERN

Figure 11 – *Circles of Concern and Influence*

140

a stressor. Your habit may be to be emotionally reactive. Don't worry, you aren't doomed. As soon as you are aware of this behavior, change it immediately. Do these things to…

Stay in your circle of influence
1. Identify the stressor.
2. Determine if it, or any part of it, is within your Circle of Influence.
3. Focus on what is within your Circle of Influence.
4. Think carefully about what things you might do to resolve the stressor.
5. Choose the behavior that you think is best.
6. Do it!

Good Self-Care…

The more you practice these steps, the easier it will be to be proactive. You won't find yourself eating to try to cope with an unresolved stressor and your bad feelings about it.

GOOD SELF-CARE…

Being self-responsible and proactive will help us significantly reduce our stress. However, there are times when our stressors cannot easily or quickly be resolved. When this happens, our bodies will physiologically be in a prolonged state of preparation for fight or flight. Emotionally, our bad feelings may dominate our lives.

In reaction to prolonged stress, you may be tempted to eat. But that will only sabotage your weight goal. Within your Circle of Influence is the choice of engaging in good self-care. Good self-care means to choose behavior that reduces the negative effect stress has on your body and your emotions.

Good self-care behaviors that will reduce the negative effects of stress on your body include exercise and eating a healthy diet. In addition, it includes practicing stress reduction techniques such as rhythmic breathing, guided imagery, and progressive relaxation.

Earlier we discussed the fact that the body produces a natural chemical of well-being called endorphins. Endorphins are released into the body when we do aerobic exercise. Rhythmic breathing will also release endorphins into your system to help you relax. To relax and release endorphins into your system do the following…

Rhythmic breathing exercise
1. Inhale through your nose as you mentally count to four.
2. Hold your breath as you count to four.
3. Exhale through your mouth as your count to six or eight.

Breathe in this manner for two to five minutes. Be sure your counting is paced so that your breathing is comfortable and easy. The more you practice this pattern, the more you will benefit from it.

Guided imagery is a process by which you take a mental vacation from your worries and concerns. In your mind you travel to a place where you can picture enjoying yourself. You might go for a mental walk on the beach or in the mountains. You might mentally go sailing or scuba diving. You might picture yourself in a place where you feel safe, secure, and free from all concern. To engage in guided imagery…

Guided imagery exercise
1. Sit in a comfortable place where you can be free from interruption.
2. Close your eyes and let your breathing be comfortable and easy.
3. Let your mind take you to a special place. Allow yourself to be fully engaged in all the sights, sounds, smells, feelings and experiences you might enjoy there.
4. Relax for as long as you choose. When it is time to reconnect with the present, slowly let your mind bring you back to where you are.
5. Take some deep breaths, open your eyes, stretch, and resume your activity.

Some people enhance their guided imagery experience by playing instrumental music softly in the background. Others play nature sounds like the sound of the sea. Many find the "white noise" produced by a fan helps them tune out awareness of any environmental noise that might disrupt their relaxation experience.

Progressive relaxation is a technique used to relax muscles that are tense due to the flight or fight response. Your muscles contract in preparation to fight or run. They remain contracted until the action of flight or fight is completed. Progressive relaxation involves gently contracting or tensing your muscles to the point at which they can no longer remain contracted and must relax. To practice progressive relaxation...

Progressive relaxation exercise

1. Sit comfortably in a place where you will not be interrupted. Close your eyes and let your breathing be easy and relaxed.
2. One by one focus on each major muscle group of your body (head, neck, shoulders, arms, hands, chest, abdomen, buttocks, legs, and feet). Tense or contract the muscles in one group as tightly as you can as you count to five. At five, let the tension go and move on to another muscle group.
3. When you have tensed and relaxed each muscle group, tense your whole body. Count to five and let the tension go.
4. Relax for as long as you like. You might choose to do some guided imagery while you relax.
5. When you are ready to end your relaxation session, slowly move and stretch your body. Take some deep breaths. Open your eyes. Continue your activity.

As with guided imagery, playing instrumental music or nature sounds or using white noise may enhance your relaxation experience.

Following weight loss surgery, some people find that their stomachs are queasy when they are stressed. Rather than wanting to eat, they avoid food. While it is a good idea not to force food on a queasy stomach, adequate food and water for the health of the body should be consumed. If you have a queasy stomach in response to stress, do not eat solid foods. Instead, consume liquid or soft foods and drink plenty of water. Doing one of the three stress management techniques described above before eating may help you to eat more comfortably.

Good
Self-Care...

In addition to these stress management techniques, many people have benefited from forms of self-care such as…

- Taking a bubble bath
- Having a manicure or pedicure
- Writing in a journal
- Talking to a friend
- Watching a funny movie
- Taking a nap
- Taking a walk in a pretty environment (park, lovely neighborhood or beach)
- Doing a craft or project
- Gardening
- Playing a game

Any activity that nurtures you and allows you to take a mental or emotional break from your stress (without eating or engaging in another self-defeating behavior) is good for you and your weight loss or maintenance program.

WHEN STRESS MANAGEMENT TECHNIQUES ARE NOT ENOUGH…

From time to time we all experience situations in which we are treated unfairly, victimized, or abused. No matter how faithfully we practice being self-responsible and proactive, or use our stress management techniques, we continue to feel overwhelmed, out of control, and emotionally distressed. In response to these situations, old habits emerge. We find ourselves engaging in self-defeating behaviors such as stress induced eating. These old habits can sabotage our weight loss and maintenance goals.

At these times, it is important to realize that the problem may not be within our Circle of Influence. It may be that the situation is unworkable or toxic. An unworkable or toxic situation is one that does not respond to our best efforts to make it better or to cope with it. It is one in which there is no possible end to the stress we experience. Instead, it will indefinitely hurt us and undermine our physical or emotional health.

If this is the case, the best way to relieve the stress and take good care of ourselves is to get away from the situation. To remain in the unworkable or toxic situation is to expose ourselves to stress that is like a poison. If we remain in such a situation, we can only experience further physical and emotional harm.

If you feel your best efforts to cope with a situation are not working but you are unsure if it is within your Circle of Influence, consultation with a trusted friend, physician or psychotherapist may be beneficial. With help you can determine the facts and make an action plan for bringing an end to the stress, or leaving it. If you must leave, encourage yourself by remembering that no job, relationship, or situation is worth the loss of your physical and emotional health.

After careful review of the situation, you may decide that change is possible or that there will be an end to the stress sometime in the future. In this case, continued support by family, friends and/or a psychotherapist can help you through. Your physician can determine if medication is needed to protect your physical and/or emotional health. A dietitian may design a special dietary program that can protect your physical health and support your weight goals.

GETTING A LIFE...

In the section of this chapter about what stress is, we indicated that stress can be having too little to do as well as having too much to do. Many severely obese people have physical illnesses or disabilities that make it impossible for them to work or to participate in the normal activities of life. They are confined to their homes with little to do but watch television and eat. Of course, the more sedentary they are and the more they snack out of loneliness, frustration, and boredom, the fatter they become. These behaviors often exacerbate physical illnesses and disabilities.

Weight loss surgeries are wonderful tools to help these people limit their eating, lose some weight, and improve their physical health. Many times, health is so improved that they can return to work and participate in all the other activities that make for a normal life. However, if that does not happen or until it does, they must assume the self-responsibility of getting a life. If you find yourself in this situation, there are several things you can do…

Tips for getting a life

1. Turn off the television. Television, especially daytime television, is not helpful to your weight loss and maintenance goals. Many commercials are for food. Most programs focus on the trials and tribulations of living. Programs that are negative in content and commercials featuring food can stimulate you to eat.

2. Get out of the house everyday. If you can walk, do so. If you can't do much walking but can drive, take yourself out somewhere. You don't have to spend money. You can go to a park, to the beach, to the library, or to visit a friend.

3. Have some social contact everyday. Make sure you see and/or talk to someone every day. Try to have social contact that is fun and uplifting.

4. Learn something every day. Keep your mind interested and active.

5. Do some meaningful work everyday. Even if you cannot work at a job, there are many worthwhile things you can do. Clean out the drawers of your desk or kitchen. Make a new address and phone list. Do a craft project. Do volunteer work. Many volunteer organizations need help and have tasks that fit your abilities and skills.

There is an old saying about how idle hands do the devil's work. A life that is understimulated, undercommitted, and boring can lead a patient to engage in eating behavior that will sabotage their weight loss and maintenance goal. In contrast, a life that is stimulated by interesting people and things to do, and commitments that fit your personal needs, goals, and limitations, is nourishing and fulfilling. Such a life will support your goal of a healthy body weight and an enriched overall quality of life.

Part Three

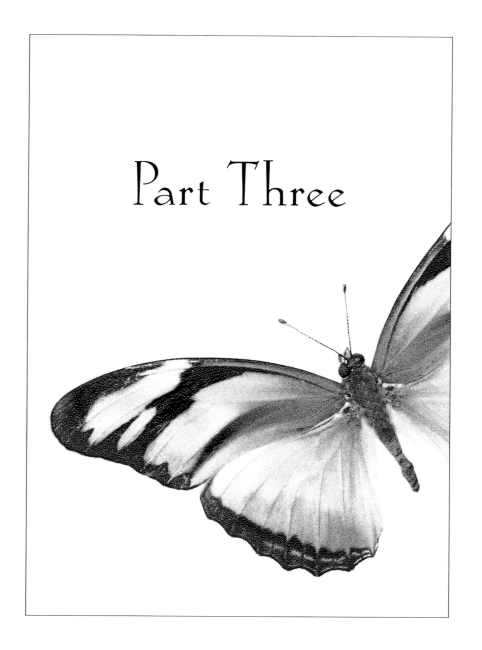

CHAPTER TEN

Living the Lighter Lifestyle

Part One and Part Two of this guide are full of valuable information. After reading them, you know what useful tools weight loss surgeries are to help those who are severely obese achieve and maintain a healthy body weight. You also know about the six important lifestyle changes that anyone wanting to achieve and maintain a healthy body weight must make.

But knowing is not enough. You, like many people, may be very knowledgeable. You may have a personal library full of information about diet and nutrition. You may know all about limiting your fat intake and how to calculate grams and calories. You may know the importance of exercise. You may even have exercise equipment in the garage and exercise videos in the closet. You may have read numerous self-help books. You may know how mismanaging your feelings, relationships, and stress may have contributed to your eating to severe obesity. But all that knowing has gotten you nowhere.

We go back to the basics. Weight loss surgeries are wonderful tools to help you achieve a healthy body weight. By using these tools, you may lose some of your excess weight. Of course, any loss is significant. But to ensure weight loss and keep it off permanently, you will also have to make the lifestyle changes described in Part Two. In addition to knowing, you must be doing.

For some, making the recommended lifestyle changes following weight loss surgery becomes easy. Weight loss surgery seems to bridge the gap between knowing and doing. For others, making the lifestyle changes remains difficult. The gap between knowing and doing remains huge. It is like standing on the North Rim of the Grand Canyon looking over to the South Rim. You know you want to get from one rim to the other, but there's all that canyon to get across. Crossing it looks to be a challenging, if not impossible, task.

Weight loss surgery gave you a tool to help you achieve and maintain a healthier weight. Perhaps all you may need to make the recommended lifestyle changes are additional tools. Tools to help you make wise nutritional choices, engage in an exercise program, develop supportive relationships, process your feelings, and effectively manage your life and stress.

Part Three is a tool kit. It contains tools in the form of lifestyle tips. As you use these tools, they can help you make the lifestyle changes you need to maximize your weight loss and life satisfaction following weight loss surgery.

Lighter Lifestyle Tip One

FOOD SHOPPING AND STORAGE

Like most people, you probably tend to eat whatever foods you find most available. If healthy foods are available, you will eat them. If not, you will eat junk foods. Eating junk foods will jeopardize your health, your weight loss, and your maintenance goal. The shopping tips below will insure that you have healthy foods available to you when it is time to eat:

Shopping Tips
1. Make a menu plan for several days or up to one week. Make a shopping list of the foods you need to buy in order to prepare the items on your menu plan.

2. At the market, buy only the foods on your list. Resolve not to fall prey to the techniques of marketing experts who tempt you to buy foods that are not on your list.
3. Shop when you feel satisfied or full. Junk food is more tempting when you are hungry.
4. Buy foods that require preparation. Self-prepared foods can be made so that they are lower in fat and calories than prepared foods. Also, you have to think twice about eating snack foods and treats if you have to prepare them rather than just stick your hand into a box or bag.
5. Shop only the aisles you need to shop. Avoid aisles with high-fat, high-calorie foods that you don't need.
6. Read labels. Some foods marked as reduced in fat or calories are still too high for a healthy diet.
7. Be honest about your purchases. Don't use the excuse that you are buying a snack or treat food for some other member of the family.
8. If you must buy snack or treat foods, buy them in individual packages so that serving sizes are limited.
9. Reward yourself for sticking to your shopping plan. *Remember*: Food is not a reward.

Everyone knows about the "see food" diet… you see food and you eat it! It seems to be a common human reaction that the sight or smell of food triggers the desire to eat. To limit your exposure to food and the temptation to eat inappropriately, store foods carefully once you get home from the market.

Storage Tips
1. Store food in containers that you cannot see through. Make sure the container seals tightly to keep tempting smells inside.
2. Store high-calorie, high-fat foods in hard to reach places. If you have an extra refrigerator or pantry in the garage or basement, put them there. If you must keep them in the house, store them in the back of the freezer or on your highest shelf.
3. Do not keep snack or treat foods on your kitchen counter or in bowls around the house.

151

Special note: Be creative in thinking about ways to store foods. One patient stored snack and treat foods in her teenage daughter's room. Her daughter was very protective of "her space" and did verbal battle with anyone who came in uninvited. It wasn't worth a fight for the patient to pursue a snack or treat.

Lighter Lifestyle Tip Two

FOOD PREPARATION AND SERVING

Eating serves so many purposes in our lives. Eating food is necessary for our physical survival and overall health. But it also has social and emotional purposes. Following weight loss surgery your challenge is to learn to prepare, serve, and eat a limited amount of food in ways that satisfy all of these purposes. Learning to prepare food in tender, tasty ways is important.

Food Preparation Tips

1. Learn to be a low-fat, low-calorie cook. Watch healthful cooking shows on television or take a cooking class. Give away your old cookbooks and replace them with low-fat, low-calorie cookbooks.
2. Make your own cookbook. Include favorite old recipes that you have adjusted to decrease the fat and calorie content. Add new low-fat, low-calorie recipes you get from support groups and other patients, or from magazines, newspapers, and cooking shows.
3. Learn to add flavor to foods with herbs and spices instead of fat.
4. Organize your kitchen so that healthful ingredients are always on hand. Throw out or give away high-fat, high-calorie ingredients you no longer need.
5. Make cooking simple. Invest in cookware and appliances that allow for low-fat food preparation. A crock pot or pressure cooker can make foods moist and tender so that they are easy to eat.
6. Make cooking and clean-up fun. Share the responsibilities with other family members. If cooking alone, chew gum or sip a non- or low-calorie beverage to keep your mouth busy and to avoid tasting or snacking.

To limit stimulation and add to the enjoyment of your meal try these...

Food Serving Tips

1. Make dining enjoyable by serving food on fun, interesting, and/or pretty china.
2. Fill plates at the stove rather than eating family style.
3. Eat in different settings; near the fireplace in the winter; on the patio in the summer.
4. Turn on some music.
5. Light some candles.
6. Turn off the television and enjoy some interesting conversation.
7. When you are finished eating, leave the table. Do additional socializing away from food.
8. When eating alone, have something interesting to do between bites (read a book or work on a puzzle). This will eliminate the temptation to eat too fast and encourage you to take the full 20 to 40 minutes of eating time that is recommended following weight loss surgery.

Special Note: One patient found it very boring to drink her protein drink regularly. She purchased some pretty crystal glasses just for drinking it and made the experience more enjoyable.

Lighter Lifestyle Tip Three

ENJOYING HOLIDAYS, PARTIES, AND RESTAURANTS

Holidays, parties, and dining at restaurants are an important part of life. After weight loss surgery you can enjoy these festive experiences and still protect your weight loss. Here are some tips for enjoying special food occasions.

Restaurants

1. Plan ahead. Consider the restaurant where you will be dining and think about what you might order when you get there. If you feel you will be tempted by high-fat, high-calorie foods, avoid looking at the menu.

2. In anticipation of your dining experience, lighten up other meals. Lighten up by decreasing calories, not by skipping meals. If you skip meals, you may find yourself so hungry you do not eat carefully enough to tolerate your food selection.

3. Order *a la carté*. An elegant appetizer and small soup or salad can make a meal special.

4. Make special requests. Many restaurants have light menu items or will prepare foods to request. Don't hesitate to ask for foods prepared "your way." Salad dressing can be served on the side and foods can be steamed, poached, or broiled instead of fried. Foods can be served without heavy sauces.

5. Monitor your portion sizes. Share a meal with someone else. Have the waiter put half of your meal into a "to go" container before serving your plate.

6. Watch alcohol intake. Alcohol contains empty calories. Many people experience a decreased tolerance to alcohol following weight loss surgery (intoxication occurs more quickly). If you wish to have an alcoholic beverage, order low-calorie drinks and have them made with lots of mixer.

7. Enjoy dessert wisely. Order dessert only if you really want it and have planned for the calories. To avoid overindulging, share a dessert. As an alternative to dessert, carry low-fat, sugar free candies or mints with you as an after meal treat.

Parties and Holidays
In addition to all of the above…

1. Consider your diet phase. Talk to your host or hostess before the event to avoid possible misunderstanding (you only need to say that you are

on a special diet for medical reasons). Offer to bring something you know you can eat.

2. Eat special foods if they fit your food phase. Skip the high-fat, high-calorie filler foods such as nuts, chips and dips.

Special Note: At special events, people are often encouraged to eat a lot of food. Many patients have developed tactics to avoid being encouraged to eat more than they want or can hold. Two tips may be useful to you. 1) Always keep a partially full glass or plate in your hand. If people see you already have something, they may not offer you more. 2) Play with your food (I know your mother told you not to do this). If you push food around on your plate now and again, you will give the appearance of eating.

Lighter Lifestyle Tip Four

COPING WITH FOOD CRAVINGS

Every day you receive many triggers to eat that are completely unrelated to the nutritional needs of your body. Triggers that encourage you to eat when you are not hungry lead to cravings for food. A craving may be triggered by a time of day, an activity, a feeling, or the smell or sight of food. If you are like most people, you most commonly crave high-fat, high-sugar foods.

The size of your stomach pouch will control how much food you can eat at one time. But it is left to you to determine when and what you will eat. If you let your cravings determine your food choices, you may eat so many high-fat, high-sugar foods that you will sabotage your weight loss or maintenance.

To help you control your cravings, do the following:

1. Identify what triggers lead to cravings. Keeping an eating diary or journal may help you do this. Write down the time of day, what is happening at that time, how you are feeling, and what food you crave. Also write down when and what you last ate and when and what you last drank.

2. If it has been a long time since your last meal, you may really be hungry. Choose to eat something nutritious. Make sure future meals are spaced so that you don't get so hungry that a craving occurs.

3. If you are thirsty, you may need to drink some water. Thirst can trigger a craving. Make sure you drink enough water to keep yourself hydrated. If possible, carry a water bottle with you at all times.

4. Check to see if you are eating nutritious foods that stick with you. If you are not, food may be emptying from the stomach pouch quickly, causing you to crave food.

5. If you do not want to give in to a craving do some exercise or distract yourself. Exercising for 10 to 20 minutes will release glucose into your system and may end your craving. Getting involved in an activity for 45 minutes may divert your attention long enough for the craving to go away.

6. If you do decide to give in to a craving, try eating a low-fat version or just a small amount of the craved food to see if that will make the craving go away. Some dietitians recommend that if you have a craving, it is best to wait until late in the day to have a small serving of the craved food. You might have a small serving of ice cream as a dessert after dinner. If you do this, you don't deprive yourself of a favorite food, but you eat it in small portions as part of your total nutritional plan. Being deprived of a favorite food may ultimately lead to a binge. Also, by eating the food as part of a meal late in the day, you won't be able to eat a large amount of it. Patients who have had a combined restrictive/malabsorptive procedure or a mainly malaborptive procedure will need to choose low or sugar-free and/or low or fat-free treat foods in order to avoid the unpleasant after-effects cause by eating these foods (dumping or diarrhea).

7. The best way to avoid food cravings is to eat a well-balanced diet and to drink plenty of water.

Special Note: In the first few weeks after surgery, some patients crave food frequently. This may be a part of the grieving process associated with major loss or change. If this is the case, working through the grieving process is the best way to deal with the cravings.

Some patients find that they lose all interest in food at some point following weight loss surgery. This loss of interest in food may be temporary or permanent. If you lose interest in food, remember that it is important to eat regularly to protect your health. You may need to develop cues to remind yourself to eat. Set the alarm on your wrist watch. When the alarm goes off, it is your cue that it is time to eat.

Lighter Lifestyle Tip Five

CHARTING YOUR PROGRESS

Like most weight loss surgery patients, you will enjoy watching your body change and charting your progress toward your goal. The best ways of doing this are weighing and measuring yourself on a regular schedule. It is important, however, to have a sensible schedule for weighing and measuring yourself so that you are encouraged, not discouraged, by what the scale and the tape measure show you.

To make sure your weight and measurement plan is sensible include the following…

1. Establish a regular frequency for weighing and measuring yourself. Once a week, or once a month, is good. Weighing or measuring yourself more than once a week is too much. Record your progress.
2. Weigh and measure yourself at the same time of day. Choose morning or evening, but don't vary the two.
3. Weigh or measure yourself in similar clothing… or lack of it.
4. Expect variation in the rate of weight or inches lost. Don't expect to lose the same amount from week to week or month to month.
5. Don't panic over small gains or increases. All people experience fluctuations in their weight. It is also important to remember the body's oxidation process for getting rid of fat. During weight loss, fat is broken down into carbon dioxide and water. The body gets rid of the carbon

dioxide quickly as we exhale. The water must travel through the body to the kidneys. Water weighs more than fat and may result in some bloating or weight gain until the water is excreted through urination. Women must also consider their normal menstrual cycle. If you gained weight during your period before weight loss surgery, most likely you will continue to do so after surgery.

Lighter Lifestyle Tip Six

OVERCOMING PLATEAUS

Immediately following weight loss surgery, you may lose both pounds and inches rapidly. Sooner or later, however, the rate of pounds and inches being lost will slow down. This is a natural body process. For overall health, it is better to lose weight and inches gradually rather than quickly.

At some point on your weight loss program, the rate of pounds and inches lost may stop completely. This, too, is a natural process and is called a plateau. A plateau is the way your body adjusts to the chemical and biological changes occurring during weight loss.

Plateaus are inevitable and should be taken in stride. They are not a sign that you have lost all the weight you can or that you will begin to regain weight. However, if a plateau continues for more than a few weeks, it will be important to do one or more of the following:

1. Check your nutritional program. Are you following the nutrition plan carefully? Have you kept your calorie intake to a weight loss level? Are you eating a nutritionally balanced diet? If not, your body may choose not to lose weight.
2. Check your exercise program. Are you being consistent in the amount of exercise you are doing? If you have decreased the amount, frequency, or intensity of exercise, your body may slow or stop it's burning of fat.
3. Have you added muscle building exercises to your program? If so, you may have built enough muscle to offset the loss of fat. Remember

muscle weighs more than fat and may slow or temporarily stop weight loss. However, you should still be losing inches.

4. If you are following your nutritional and exercise program faithfully, you may temporarily need to decrease your calorie intake and/or increase the amount of exercise you are doing to start weight loss again. Check with your physician, or an appropriate support team member, for some recommendations on the best ways to use this method of ending a plateau.

5. If you have been on the weight loss phase of your program for several months, you may need to consult with your physician or support team members about temporarily increasing your calorie intake. When your body has been losing a lot of weight, it may need to take a "rest" from the calorie restriction imposed by the diet. Your physician or support team members can help you make wise decisions about how much and the best way to increase your calorie intake.

Lighter Lifestyle Tip Seven

RECOVERING FROM NUTRITIONAL SLIPS

The idea that you can and should live a perfect life is a myth… it is an impossibility. But many weight loss surgery patients expect themselves to be perfect when it comes to a diet program. They believe they are on a diet when they are following their nutritional plan perfectly. The are off a diet if they slip from the plan even once, or in some minor way.

In addition, when they are not perfect in following a nutritional plan, they view themselves as bad, weak, or unworthy of success. This viewpoint has often led them to persist in poor eating behavior when they slipped off their program. They do this because they think, "If I do not follow my dietary program perfectly, I am a failure. Since I cannot follow my program perfectly and I will fail, I might as well not even try to lose weight."

The truth is that all people make unwise food choices from time to time. Instead of wasting energy punishing yourself, get back on track immediately. Here are some things you can do to recover from nutritional slips…

1. Forgive yourself for being human.
2. Start eating wisely immediately. Don't decide to wait until tomorrow to get back on track and allow yourself to continue making poor food choices today.
3. Ask yourself if there is something you can learn about yourself through the nutritional slip. What high risk situations or triggers might be tempting you? Make a plan to deal with them better in the future.
4. Ask yourself if there are any feelings you are trying to avoid or "stuff down" by eating. If so, face them and work them through.
5. Lighten up on the calorie content of your meals, and/or increase your exercise, in order to decrease the possibility of slowing your weight loss or of experiencing weight regain following a slip.
6. Seek help and support if you need it. Remember, successful dieters don't go it alone.

Lighter Lifestyle Tip Eight

SETTING GOALS FOR SUCCESS

Success in achieving and maintaining your goal weight following weight loss surgery will require you to make changes in one or more of these areas: Your diet, physical activity level, attitudes, relationships, and stress management skills. Like weight loss, lifestyle changes don't happen magically. They take commitment and determination.

A good way to make change is to set a goal. Many people set goals in the same way that they make New Year's resolutions. They are great ideas that never become realities. To help your goals become realities do the following:

Goal Setting Tips
1. Select one thing you would like to change. State your goal in a simple sentence. *Example:* I want to make exercise a regular part of my life.

2. Write down all the reasons why it is important for you to achieve this goal. *Example:* To lose weight more quickly; to tone and firm my muscles; to decrease the appearance of flab; to feel better; to increase my stamina.

3. Make an action plan for achieving your goal. An action plan defines what you are going to do and when you are going to do it. *Example:* In one month, I want to be walking for one hour four times each week. I will arrange my schedule so that I can walk on Monday, Wednesday, Friday and Saturday. I will walk while my family is eating dinner and washing the dinner dishes. I will begin by walking for ten minutes and will gradually increase my walking time to one hour by the end of the month.

4. Make a chart for your progress. *Example:* Post a calendar where you will see it often (your bathroom mirror, your clothes closet door). Highlight the days you plan to walk. When you walk, mark off the days in some way (use happy faces or fun stickers).

5. Plan a reward for your efforts. *Example:* Put $1.00 in a kitty each time you walk. You get all the money to spend in any way you would like when the month is up. Plan a special activity or purchase for when the month is out and you have reached your goal. You might have a manicure or pedicure. You might go to a play or museum. You might buy a book or an item of clothing or jewelry.

Special Note: Two additional factors are important to goal setting. 1) Make sure your goal is reasonable. Your goal is reasonable if you can accomplish it with whatever time, energy, personal or interpersonal limitations you have. If you have one hundred pounds to lose, an impossible goal is to lose it all in three months! 2) Some people need negative consequences to keep them working on their goal. A negative consequence is something you don't want to do, but must, if you do not work toward or accomplish your goal. Using the example given above, a negative consequence might be having to wash the family dinner dishes if you don't walk on the days you have scheduled to walk. Or, it might be choosing an exercise monitor to whom you will have to pay $1.00 each time you do not walk.

Setting Goals
for Success

Lighter Lifestyle Tip Nine

MOTIVATING YOURSELF FOR SUCCESS

When starting any new program or project, our motivation is high. We are enthusiastic, positive, and eager to go. Sooner or later, our motivation usually wanes. This often happens when it takes a long time to reach our goal, or when it is more difficult to achieve our goal than we thought it would be.

Weight loss surgeries are wonderful tools to help you accomplish your goal of losing weight and of improving your health and quality of life. But it will take time to reach your goal. Sometimes living the lifestyle you need to live to support weight loss and maintenance will be difficult. Here are some tips to help keep your motivation up.

Good Ways to Motivate Yourself

1. Make a chart on which you record each step of your progress… no matter how small that step may be. Read your chart when you are feeling down. Examples: I can breathe more easily; my sleep has improved; I can walk without pain; I can sit down in the bathtub; I can see my toes; I can buy clothes in a regular department store or boutique; I no longer need insulin for diabetes; I can zip up my pants without lying on the bed and tugging at the zipper; I am down (number) dress, shirt, or pants sizes.

2. Celebrate each success with a reward… no matter how small the success or how small the reward.

3. Make a collage illustrating all of the things you look forward to having or doing when you reach your goal.

4. Put motivational statements and affirmations around where you can see them frequently.

5. Keep a progress bulletin board, photo album, or video. Examples: Take pictures of yourself each month to see how you are changing. Keep the largest pair of pants you ever wore. Try them on to see how baggy they are getting. Each month or two, take a picture of yourself wearing the baggy pants. Post the pictures to help you visualize and internalize your progress.

162

Special Note: The husband of one patient wanted to practically support his wife toward her weight loss goal. He decided upon some rewards he would give to her and wrote them on small pieces of paper. Each time his wife accomplished a goal that deserved recognition; he let her pick one piece of paper. He gave her the reward written on the paper she chose. A very nice idea!

Lighter Lifestyle Tip Ten

FINDING SOLUTIONS TO PROBLEMS

Say the word problem and most of us have an immediate intellectual and emotional response. Intellectually we equate the word problem with a challenge, difficulty, perplexity, or vexation. Something that we don't want that is getting in the way of something we do want. Emotionally we experience a problem as a feeling of being distressed, sad, mad, or scared. Something that makes us feel bad.

Situations that make us feel bad often lead us to engage in self-defeating behavior to try to distract ourselves from the problem, or to soothe away our bad feelings. Some people drink alcoholic beverages to avoid problems and the bad feelings they bring. Others shop or engage in recreational activities. You may have eaten to distract yourself, or to soothe away your bad feelings, when you had a problem. After repeatedly eating over problems, you know distraction and soothing with food is not an effective way to get rid of them. It simply does not work.

What does work? Solving a problem so that you are no longer challenged, perplexed, or vexed. Solving it so that you feel glad instead of bad. The steps below can help you solve problems and feel glad.

Steps That Solve Problems
  1. Identify what situation is a problem to you right now.
  2. Write down how you feel about it.
  3. What would you like the situation to be so that you can feel glad?

4. What part of the situation fits within your Circle of Influence? What part fits within your Circle of Concern?
5. Focus only on that part of the situation that fits within your Circle of Influence.
6. Write down all the possible ways you might respond to the problem so that it is solved. Which one(s) would help the situation be like you would want it to be and help you feel glad?
7. Choose a solution and try it out.
8. If your first choice doesn't work, repeat step 7. Be persistent. Most likely, by being persistent, you will find a solution that does work and that helps you feel glad.
9. If you just cannot find a solution on your own, get help. Sometimes we are so involved in a problem that we just cannot see an answer. A trusted family member or friend may provide us with a new perspective to the problem that will lead to a solution.
10. When the problem is solved, congratulate yourself. You did well! Now go about your day feeling glad (and with a little more self-confidence and self-esteem)!

Special Note: By using the steps above, most of the problems of everyday living can be solved. It would be dishonest, however, to say that they can all be solved. Sometimes a life circumstance or problem is firmly rooted in our Circle of Concern and we have little, if any, influence upon it.

When we cannot solve a problem and must live with continuing feelings of sadness, anger, or fear, we must engage in good self-caring behavior. Instead of returning to old eating behaviors, it would be better for you to seek support and guidance from family, friends, your physician or a psychotherapist. It would help you to process and work through the distressing feelings you feel about the problem. It would also be good for you to engage in some stress reduction exercises to relax your body and your mind.

Lighter Lifestyle Tip Eleven

TAKING CHARGE OF YOUR TIME

Time is a necessary resource you will need in order to make the many lifestyle changes necessary to achieve and maintain a healthy body weight. You will need time to change your cooking and eating behavior. You will need time to exercise. You will need time to attend classes and a support group. Finding the time to do these things may seem impossible. Most weight loss surgery patients already have very active lives trying to juggle the demands of work, family, friends, home responsibilities, and more.

If we are honest with ourselves, however, we waste more time than we care to admit. We can live a lighter lifestyle, if we are willing to take charge of how we spend our time. Below are some guidelines for taking charge of your time so that you will have the time you need to spend on your weight loss and maintenance program.

Making Time

1. For one week (or a longer period, if you choose), don't change a thing. Instead, carry around a notebook and write down everything you do and how much time it takes.
2. Sit down in a quiet place and carefully analyze how you spend your time. Group activities into categories. You might have categories for Job, Housekeeping, Family, Paperwork, and Recreation.
3. Identify those areas where your time is used well and those where you really do waste it.
4. Make an action plan for taking charge of your time.
   - List the activities that are essential for living and how much time they take.
   - Note the activities you must do yourself.
   - Note any activities that you can delegate to others or shorten the time you spend on them.

- Resolve to give up perfectionism. Determine not to waste time trying to do everything just right - as if you were trying to impress some special guest. Just do some things good enough.
- List those activities that waste your time. Resolve to cut back on the amount of time you give them or eliminate them altogether.

5. Reassess. How much time have you found by doing this exercise?
6. Make an action plan to use this time to support your weight loss program and/or to do other things of more importance to you.
   - Schedule time for exercise.
   - Schedule time for relaxation.
   - Schedule time to attend a class or support group.
   - Use any remaining time to enrich your personal life and your relationships.
7. Use the tips for successful goal setting to help you achieve your goal of taking charge of your time.

Special Note: There will always be situations in life that take away our choice about how we spend our time. We might have a rush job at work or our child may be sick. Situations such as these are to be expected and we must respond to them. As soon as the special circumstance is over, determine to get back on track with your action plan for using your time to support your weight and health goals. Don't let the situation permanently derail you!

Lighter Lifestyle Tip Twelve

ASSERTIVE COMMUNICATION

Those who are the most successful in reaching their goal weight, have help from their families and friends. It is unrealistic to believe that family members and friends automatically know what to do to be supportive. If they are left to figure it out on their own, they may do the wrong things.

If you want your family members and friends to help you by doing things that are supportive, you need to tell them what to do to be helpful. You need to tell them what not to do. You need to negotiate necessary behavioral and lifestyle change. And you need to confront behavior that hurts or sabotages you. The best way to do this is through assertive communication.

You are being assertive when you express your true feelings and needs and do not let others take advantage of you. Being assertive also means being considerate of the feelings and needs of others and not trying to take advantage of them. When you are assertive, you can act in your own best interest without feeling that you have done something wrong or bad. By being considerate of others, you can usually get what you want without hurting others or making them angry with you.

Tips for Assertive Communication
1. Identify what you need to talk about. *Example:* I need to attend my weight loss education and support class on Tuesday nights from 6:30 to 7:30. I need my husband to watch the children, feed them dinner, and get them ready for bed.
2. Arrange a time to talk. *Example:* "I need to talk to you about attending my class. Is this a good time? If not now, when would be a good time?"
3. Discuss your need or situation clearly, including the specifics about time, place, and frequency and what you need from the other person. *Example:* "It is very important to my successful weight loss following weight loss surgery that I attend the weekly education and support class. The class meets every Tuesday evening from 6:30 to 7:30. It is recommended that I attend for one year and I would like to attend as frequently as I can. To attend, I need your help. I need you to watch the children on Tuesday evenings, feed them dinner, and get them ready for bed. Is that workable for you?"
4. Listen calmly to the reply. *Example:* No faces or noises.
5. If the answer is yes, show your appreciation. *Example:* "Thanks honey. I really appreciate your help (hugs and kisses)."
6. If the answer is no, then pursue another solution. *Example:* "I'm disappointed. It is really important to me to attend the class and I will feel

hurt and angry if I don't. I will arrange for child care for the children so that I can attend."

7. If the answer is something like, "You know that I like to go to the gym on Tuesday evenings," negotiate. *Example:* "That's right. I know going to the gym is important to you. Can you do it another night. I would be glad to (take over some responsibility) so you could."

8. If you have to negotiate or find another solution, be graceful. Don't pout, yell, or punish. Gracious behavior may contribute to getting what you want the next time.

Special Note: The words above are rather formal in order to make the example clear. What is more important than the specific words are the attitudes you project. It is important to project an attitude of respect for your own needs. It is important to project an attitude of respect for the needs of the other person. It is also important to project a win-win, rather than a win-lose, attitude. In other words, you have reached a win-win solution when both people feel good about the way the situation is resolved. If you have trouble being assertive… you are usually too passive or aggressive in your communication style… an assertiveness training class or self-help book might be useful.

Lighter Lifestyle Tip Thirteen

PROCESSING YOUR FEELINGS

Many people engage in self-defeating behaviors, such as overeating, to try to avoid, stuff-down, or soothe away uncomfortable feelings. While eating may be comforting for a short while, it does not take care of the feelings. When emotional eating stops, we are left with the uncomfortable feeling we were eating about, plus the physical and emotional discomfort of overeating.

David Viscott, MD, described the kinds of uncomfortable feelings we feel as hurt, anxiety, anger, depression, and guilt. Hurt is what we feel when we experience a loss. Anxiety is what we feel when we anticipate a loss. Anger is what we feel when we resent a loss. Depression is what we feel when we are depleted by our loss. Guilt is what we feel when we internalize our anger and feel worthless because of the loss.

Dr. Viscott believed that if we will work through our hurt when it occurs, then, for the most part, we can avoid anxiety, anger, depression, and guilt. If we are feeling anxious, angry, depressed, or guilty, we can resolve these feelings by working through the original hurt that caused them.

Working through Hurt

1. Acknowledge and feel your hurt. *Example:* I feel hurt. It hurts (a little to a lot).
2. Identify the event, statement, and situation that hurt you. *Example:* I feel hurt because (someone said or did something hurtful).
3. If possible, communicate that hurt to the offending party. *Example:* "I feel hurt because you (be specific about what was said or done)."
4. Give the offending person a chance to reconsider what they have done. *Example:* "I don't understand or I am not comfortable with this state-ment (or behavior). Please clarify what you mean (or did)."
5. Reach an understanding with the offending person to help you resolve the hurt.
6. Forgive the person for hurting you as a sign you have let go of the pain.
7. If the other person hurt you on purpose and will not work to resolve the issue, forgive the other person anyway (this is so you can let go of the hurt). If necessary, get some distance from the person or situation so that you won't continue to be hurt.

Special Note: Sometimes we cannot resolve the hurtful issue directly with the person who hurt us. This may be because the person is no longer avail-able to talk with. Or it can be because the hurt was caused by a situation or life circumstance, not a person. This is true in the case of any hurt you feel about losing the ability to eat what and when you want to eat following weight loss surgery.

A creative way of working through this hurt is to write a goodbye letter to food. In your letter you can describe the important role food has played in your life. Write about how food has helped and/or hurt you. Describe any additional feelings such as anxiety, anger, or guilt. Forgive the food for how it has hurt you. Say goodbye. Affirm the fact that you are moving on to a healthier, happier life with a new, appropriate relationship with food.

Lighter Lifestyle Tip Fourteen

EXERCISE IN RELAXATION

Stress is an everyday experience of life. When we experience stress, our muscles tense. Progressive relaxation is an exercise that helps to reduce the tension of the muscles. Combining guided imagery with progressive relaxation can relax our mind and significantly decrease our physical and emotional experience of stress.

For maximum relaxation and enjoyment, you might want to tape this exercise so that you can play it and follow the directions. If you tape it, read the script slowly, allowing plenty of time to do each part of the exercise.

Exercise in Guided Imagery with Progressive Relaxation
I get myself comfortable. I close my eyes. I let my attention focus on my breathing. I allow my breathing to be slow, natural, and peaceful. In my mind's eye, I see myself driving in my car. I am driving away from all the pressures of my everyday environment. I am driving further and further into the country toward mountains. Fewer and fewer cars are on the road. I am finally alone and very near the mountains. I find a place to park my car and get out. I stand and look at everything around me. I notice all the sights, smells, sounds, and the feel of this mountain environment. I feel calm, peaceful, and relaxed.

I notice a stream flowing a short distance away. I walk toward the stream. As I approach, the sound of the water flowing across the rocks in the stream becomes louder and louder. It is a comforting sound. I select a place to sit down by the stream. I let the sound of the stream and the beauty of the environment help me to feel even more relaxed, peaceful, and calm.

In my mind I think about all the hassles and troubles of my daily life. One by one, my troubles become like colorful leaves that fall into the stream. I watch them drift away in the current of the water, further and further out of sight, and then be gone. I lie back on the ground and become aware of my body.

I think about my head and all the muscles in my head, neck and face. I tense all the muscles of my face until I feel them tight. I relax my face and notice the difference between how my face feels when it is tensed and when it is relaxed. I repeat the process.

I notice my shoulders, upper back, and upper chest. I tense all the muscles in these areas of my body. I hold the tension as tightly as I can. I relax the tension. As with my face, I notice the difference between the feeling of tension and relaxation. I repeat the process.

I notice my hands and arms. I tense all the muscles in my hands and arms as tightly as I can. I hold this tension. I relax. I notice the difference in the feelings. I repeat this process. I give my entire body a chance to relax.

I now notice my lower back, my lower abdomen, and my buttocks. I tense all the muscles in these areas of my body. I hold the tension. I relax. I notice the difference in the feelings. I repeat this process.

I notice my legs and feet. I tense all the muscles in my legs and feet as tightly as I can. I hold the tension. I relax. I notice the difference and repeat the process.

I now focus on my whole body. I tense my whole body as tightly as I can. I hold the tension. I relax. I notice the difference in the feelings. I repeat the process.

I am now feeling as relaxed, peaceful, and calm as I can be at this time. I enjoy the feeling. I allow my mind to refocus on the beauty of the mountain environment as long as I would like.

When I am ready, I begin to move and stretch my body. I take some deep breaths. I open my eyes. I feel relaxed, calm, and peaceful. I know I can return to my special place to relax any time I would like to do so.

Special Note: For an even more relaxing experience, you may want to do this exercise more gradually. If you do, tense and release one body part at a time (such as your face, neck, hand, arm, foot, or leg) rather than a group of body parts (face and neck, hand and arm, food and leg).

Living the Lighter Lifestyle

Closing Thoughts

Research suggests that the causes of obesity may be 50 to 70% genetic and/or hormonal. New treatments—including additional surgeries, improvements to existing surgeries and less invasive surgical methods—are likely on the horizon. While these are important, the lifestyle changes necessary to achieve and maintain weight loss are equally important. Successful weight management will always require healthy eating, regular activity and managing challenging life circumstances, thoughts, and feelings without overeating. It is my hope that the information provided in this book—along with your weight loss surgery—will enable you to live a lighter lifestyle for a lifetime.

—*Gaye Andrews, PH D, LMFT*

Recommended Reading

Many weight loss surgery patients ask for a list of books they can read to support them in living a lighter lifestyle. The books below have been helpful and inspirational to me and many patients, too. The books have been selected because they provide information important to developing the lifestyle habits necessary to successful weight loss and maintenance.

EATING FOR LIVING A LIGHTER LIFESTYLE

Albers, Susan, PSY D. *Eating Mindfully.*
   New Harbinger Publications, Inc., 2003

Bricklin, Mark. *Lose Weight Naturally.*
   MFJ Books, 1989.

Koenig, Karen R., LISCW, M ED, *The Rules of "Normal" Eating.*
   Gurze Books, 2005.

Minirth, Frank PH D, et al. *Love Hunger: Recovery From Food Addiction.*
   Thomas Nelson Publishers, 1990.

Minirth, Frank PH D, et al. *Love Hunger: Weight-loss Workbook.*
   Thomas Nelson Publishers, 1991.

Prochaska, James O., PH D, et al., *Changing for Good.*
   Quill, 2002.

EXERCISE FOR LIVING A LIGHTER LIFESTYLE

Any of the six books above.

ATTITUDES FOR LIVING A LIGHTER LIFESTYLE:

Larkey, Jan. *Flatter Your Figure*. Prentice Hall Press, 1991.

Stoddard, Alexandra. *Living A Beautiful Life*. Random House, 1986.

Stoddard, Alexandra. *Daring To Be Yourself*. Avon Nonfiction, 1990.

Stoddard, Alexandra. *Making Choices*. William Morrow and Company, 1994.

Stoop, Jan and David. *Saying Goodbye To Disappointments*. Thomas Nelson Publishers, 1993.

Walas, Kathleen. *Real Beauty… Real Women*. Master Media Limited, 1992.

NUTRITION FOR LIVING A LIGHTER LIFESTYLE

Any of the six books listed in Eating For Living A Lighter Lifestyle.

Piscatella, Joseph C. *Controlling Your Fat Tooth*. Workman Publishing, 1991.

Rosso, Julee. *Great Good Food*. Crown Publishers, Inc., 1993.

RELATIONSHIPS FOR LIVING A LIGHTER LIFESTYLE

Beattie, Melody. *Codependent No More*. Harper/Hazelden, 1987.

Buhler, Rich. *Pain And Pretending*. Thomas Nelson Publishers, 1991.

Recommended Reading

Gray, John. *Men Are From Mars, Women Are From Venus.*
Harper Collins Publishers, 1991.

Stoddard, Alexandra. *Living Beautifully Together.* Doubleday, 1989.

STRESS MANAGEMENT FOR LIVING A LIGHTER LIFESTYLE

Davis, Martha; Matthew McKay; Elizabeth Robbins Eshelman. *The Relaxation And Stress Reduction Workbook.* New Harbinger Publications, 1980.

Feldmeth, Joanne Ross; Midge Wallace Finley, *We Weep For Ourselves And Our Children.* Harper San Francisco, 1973, 1978, 1984.

Jaffee, Dennis T.; Cynthia D. Scott. *From Burnout To Balance.* McGraw Hill, 1984.

Lerner, Harriet Goldhor. *The Dance Of Anger.* Harper and Row Publishers, 1986.

Lerner, Harriet Goldhor. *The Dance Of Intimacy.* Harper and Row Publishers, 1989.

Sonkin, Daniel Jay. *Wounded Boys Heroic Men.* Longmeadow Publishers, 1992.

Stuart, Richard B.; Barbara Jacobson. *Weight, Sex And Marriage.* W.W. Norton and Company, 1987.

Recommended Reading

*Recommended
Reading*

References

ARTICLES

"Dolly: How She Lost It And Kept It Off," *First*, June 28, 1993.

"Fat Like Me, Leslie Lampert," *Ladies Home Journal*, May 1993.

"For A Lifelong Healthy Heart: Choose Exercise," James M. Rippe, MD, n.p. n.d.

Boykin, Mary Reese. "I have lost 343 pounds," Voices: A Forum For Community Issues, *Los Angeles Times*, 20 November, 1999

Gibbs, W. Wayt. "Gaining on Fat," *Scientific American*, August 1996

Stern, Judith S., SC D. "Lose The Weight – Win The Battle," *First*, June 28, 1993

Travis, John. "The Hunger Hormone?," *Science News Online, The Weekly Newsmagazine of Science*, February 16, 2002.

U.S. Department of Agriculture and the U.S. Department of Health and Human Services. "Food Guide Pyramid, a Guide to Daily Food Choices," Provided by the Education Department of the National Live Stock and Meat Board, 1993.

BOOKS

American Society for Bariatric Surgery. *Surgery For Morbid Obesity: What Patients Should Know*. American Society for Bariatric Surgery, 2000

References

BioEnterics Corporation. *A Surgical Aid In The Treatment Of Morbid Obesity: Lap-Band Adjustable Gastric Banding System Information For Patients*. BioEnterics Corporation, 2001.

Bricklin, Mark. *Lose Weight Naturally*. MJF Books, 1989.

Covey, Stephen R. *The Seven Habits Of Highly Effective People*. Simon and Schuster; 1989.

Crenshaw, Roger T. MD; Theresa L. Crenshaw, MD. *Expressing Your Feelings*. Roger Crenshaw, 1982.

Davis, McKay, Eshelman. *The Relaxation and Stress Reduction Workbook*. New Harbinger Publications, 1980.

Deitel, Mervyn. *Surgery for the Morbidly Obese Patient*, FD-Communications Inc.; 1989, 1998.

Genton, Marie. *The Dumping Syndrome: A Support Group Special Presentation*, Brotman Medical Center, June 22, 2000.

Goble, Frank G. *The Third Force: The Psychology Of Abraham Maslow*. Washington Square Press, 1970.

Herbert, Victor, MD, FACP; Genell J. Subak-Sharpe, MS. *Total Nutrition: The Only Guide You'll Ever Need*. New York: St. Martin's Griffith, 1995.

Kiester, Edwin Jr. ed. *New Family Medical Guide*. Better Homes and Gardens Books, 1982.

180

Miller, Benjamin F., MD. *The Complete Medical Guide.*
   Simon and Schuster, 1978.

Minirth, Frank PH D, et al. *Love Hunger: Recovery From Food Addiction.*
   Thomas Nelson Publishers, 1990.

Minirth, Frank PH D, et al. *Love Hunger: Weight-loss Workbook.*
   Thomas Nelson Publishers, 1991.

Mosby. *Mosby's Pocket Dictionary Of Medicine, Nursing, & Allied Health,
   Third Edition.* Mosby, A Harcourt Health Sciences Company, 1998.

Peck, M. Scott, MD. *The Road Less Traveled.* Simon and Schuster, 1978.

Pines, Ayala M.; Elliot Aronson; Ditsa Kafry. *Burnout: From Tedium To
   Personal Growth.* The Free Press, 1981.

Rosso, Julee. *Great Good Food: Luscious Lower-Fat Cooking.*
   Crown Publishers, Inc., 1993.

Shape Up America and American Obesity Association. *Guidance for
   Treatment of Adult Obesity.*
   Shape Up America and American Obesity Association; 1996, 1998.

Stoop, Jan and David. *Saying Goodbye To Disappointments.*
   Thomas Nelson Publishers, 1993.

Stuart, Richard B.; Barbara Jacobson; *Weight, Sex and Marriage: A
   Delicate Balance.* W. W. Norton and Company, 1987.

Viscott, David, MD. *Emotionally Free.* Contemporary Books, Inc., 1992.

Wadden, Thomas A.; Theodore B. VanItallie, ed. *Treatment of the Seriously
   Obese Patient.* The Guilford Press, New York and London, 1992.

Waterhouse, Debra, MPH, RD. *Why Women Need Chocolate.*
Hyperion, New York, 1995.

Woodward, Bryan G. MPH, LCEP. *A Complete Guide To Obesity Surgery*:
*Everything You Need To Know About Weight Loss Surgery And How To
Succeed.* LifeLong Bariatrics, LLC, in cooperation with Trafford
Publishing, 2001.

MEDICAL PAPERS:

"Gastrointestinal Surgery For Severe Obesity," *National Institutes Of Health
Consensus Development Conference Statement*, March 25-27, 1991.

"LiteLife Dietary Program," St. Luke Medical Center, Pasadena, CA.

"SurgiSlim Diet," St. Luke Medical Center, Pasadena, CA. n.d.

Gilman, Tricia; Dale Gilman. "Living Happily and Healthily with Your
Surgery (LGB)," Santa Barbara: Gilman Enterprises, 1996.

Shamblin, James R. MD, FACS; William R. Shamblin, MD, FACS "Bariatric
Surgery Should Be More Widely Accepted," n.d.

Sugarman, Harvey J. MD; David M. Hume. "Gastric Bypass for Morbid
Obesity," *Surgical Rounds*, March 1993.

Weintraub, Michael MD, ed. "Long-term Weight Control: The National
Heart, Lung, And Blood Institute Funded Multimodal Intervention
Study," The Departments of Community And Preventative Medicine,
Pharmacology and Medicine, University of Rochester School Of
Medicine And Dentistry
13/0/36/36-412.

BariatricEdge, Ethcon Endo-Surgery, Inc. "About Morbid Obesity."
  http://www.bariatricedge.com/dtcf/pages/1_MorbidObesity.htm
  (cited August 8, 2008).

Health Grades, Minimally Invasive Bariatric Surgical Services,
  "Laparoscopic and Open Sleeve Gastrectomy."
  http://www.transmed.tv
  (cited October 18, 2008).

Laparoscopic Associates of San Fransicso (LAPSF). "Vertical Sleeve
  Gastrectomy (VSG)—Also known as Sleeve Gastrectomy, Vertical
  Gastrectomy."
  http://www.obesityhelp.com/forums/vsg/mode,pcontent/cmsID,8874/
  (cited August 8, 2008).

"Surgically Slim, Minimally Invasive Laparoscopic Procedures, Mount
  Sinai Section of Bariatric Surgery, The Vertical Sleeve Gastrectomy."
  http://www.surgicallyslim.com/sleeve.htm
  (cited August 8, 2008).

"WIN Weight-control Information Network, National Institutes of Health,
  Statistics Related to Overweight and Obesity."
  www.win.niddk.nih.gov
  (cited August 8, 2008).

References

PRESENTATIONS:

Andrews, Gaye, PH D and LeMont, Diane, PH D, "Psychosocial Issues in Weight Management: Prescriptions for Success." Paper presented at Contemporary Forums Obesity Treatment and Prevention Conferences Orlando, FL, March 27, 2008 and San Francisco, CA April 24, 2008, Contemporary Forums, Dublin, CA

References

Index

186

Goals 34, 70, 118, 136, 137, 138, 139, 144, 145, 146, 160, 166
    Sabotage of 102, 104, 107, 115, 117, 118, 122, 124, 136, 137, 141, 144, 146, 155
    Setting of 160–162
Grams 78, 149
Grhelin 5
Grief 104
Guidelines 20, 25, 26, 27, 31, 33, 41, 44, 45, 46, 47, 51, 61, 62, 64, 75–76, 80, 83, 165

H

Habits 20, 35, 41, 60, 61, 92, 144
Hair Loss 27, 48, 88
Health 1, 2, 4, 31, 32, 33, 35, 36, 45, 46, 48, 49, 70, 73, 80, 81, 83, 84, 87, 88, 91, 93,
    103, 107, 110, 115, 116, 119, 122, 124, 125, 136, 139, 143, 144, 145, 150, 152, 157,
    158, 162, 166
Heart Rate 95
Hospitalization 33, 34
Hunger 44, 45, 85, 86, 87, 88, 93
Hypertension: *See* Comorbidities

I

Ideal Body Weight (IBW) 76, 77, 78
Ileum: *See* Digestive System
Insurance 42
Iron 11, 26, 66, 83, 84

J

Jejunum: *See* Digestive System

K

L

Lactose Intolerance 27, 31, 51, 52
Laparoscopic Surgery: *See* Surgery, Methods
Large Intestine: *See* Digestive System

N

O

P

Q

R

Index

Index

T

Technical Challenge: *See* Support Groups, Important Services
Technical Support: *See* Support Groups, Important Services
Test(s) 20, 35, 84, 122
Timed-release pills: *See* Pills

U

V

Vegetables 51, 64, 65, 71, 72, 75, 79, 80, 84, 132
Vitamins 83–88
    A 26, 32, 71, 84
    B1 26, 32
    B12 11, 26, 32, 66, 83
    B6 26, 32
    C 72
    D 26, 32, 71, 72, 84
    E 26, 32, 71, 84
    K 26, 32, 71, 84
Vomiting 21, 48, 62, 64, 104

W

Water 2, 64, 70, 80, 84, 84–85, 85, 96, 115, 143, 156, 157, 158, 170, 171
Weight Loss Obstacles 102, 103, 103–105, 105, 106, 109, 123, 132, 136
Weight Plateau: *See* Plateau
Weight Watchers: *See* Support Groups
Work 33, 131, 133, 134, 145, 146, 166

X

Y

Z

Index